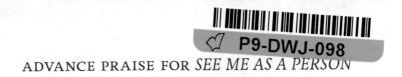
ADVANCE PRAISE FOR *SEE ME AS A PERSON*

"*See Me as a Person* is extremely well written and thought provoking. The book gives true insight on how to achieve improved patient satisfaction by enabling staff to create therapeutic relations with patients and families."

RONALD ALDRICH, LFACHE, CHAIR, BOARD OF DIRECTORS, CHRISTUS ST. VINCENT REGIONAL MEDICAL CENTER, SANTA FE, NM

"This book is easy to read and is applicable to all levels from staff to administration, providing significant information related to how to maintain high patient satisfaction scores. *See Me as a Person* provides executive leadership the clear message that scripting is not the answer to patient satisfaction. Fostering the process to see patients as people is the key, and this text helps organizations do just that."

SUSAN K. STEELE-MOSES, DNS, APRN-CNS, AOCN, RESEARCH DIRECTOR, OUR LADY OF THE LAKE REGIONAL MEDICAL CENTER, BATON ROUGE, LA

"*See Me as a Person* brings back into your hands the 'art' of medicine. The use of story was wonderful. The concepts are fundamental to human caring, but so often overlooked in the prevalent medical paradigm. We must remove the robotic, automatic, scripted responses we as caregivers have been fed and replace them with authentic caring and interest in our fellow man."

STACEY CROPLEY, DNP, RN, CPN, AUTHOR OF *THE RELATIONSHIP-BASED CARE MODEL: EVALUATION OF THE IMPACT ON PATIENT SATISFACTION, LENGTH OF STAY, AND READMISSION RATES,* JONA, 2012

"This book is the foundation from which nurses, physicians, and allied health professionals can reconnect to their meaning and purpose as caregivers. It will affirm you, reassure you, and give you a new set of tools that will enable you to build therapeutic relationships quickly and effectively, even when time is at a premium. I believe this should be required reading for every clinical and medical student."

Debra Fox, MS, RN, CNS, Chief Nursing Officer, McKee Medical Center, Loveland, CO

"*See Me as a Person* delivers the inspiration and 'how tos' to engage in a therapeutic relationship. Up until now we were telling clinicians to establish a therapeutic relationship but did not give them the recipe. Now they have the recipe."

Patricia Ritola, MSN, RN, NE-BC, Relationship-Based Care Implementation Leader, Munson Medical Center, Traverse City, MI

See me as a person

Creating therapeutic relationships with patients and their families

MARY KOLOROUTIS AND MICHAEL TROUT

Written by
Mary Koloroutis
Michael Trout

Koloroutis, Mary.
 See me as a person : creating therapeutic relationships with patients and their families / by Mary Koloroutis and Michael Trout.
        p. ; cm.
 Includes bibliographical references and index.
 ISBN 978-1-886624-83-2 (pbk. : alk. paper)
 I. Trout, Michael David. II. Title.
 [DNLM: 1. Physician-Patient Relations. 2. Nurse-Patient Relations. W 62]
  610.69'6—dc23

                                2012030753

Printed in the United States of America

First Printing: 2012

16 15 14 13 12   5 4 3 2 1

Printed in the United States of America.

Cover and interior design by James Monroe Design, LLC.

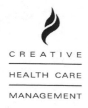

CREATIVE

HEALTH CARE

MANAGEMENT

For permission and ordering information, write to:
Creative Health Care Management, Inc.
5610 Rowland Road, Suite 100
Minneapolis, Minnesota 55343
e-mail: chcm@chcm.com
or call 800.728.7766 • 952.854.9015
www.chcm.com

Dedicated to our daughter, Alicia,
whose quest to become a caring nurse
has inspired us.

Dear Kristen,
In appreciation for your
scholarship, compassion and
leadership. We humbly
thank you.

Mary & Michael
October, 2012

Contents

Chapter Two

Presence through Attunement 59

Chapter Three

*Wondering: Cultivating Curiosity for Efficient and
Compassionate Practice* 93

Chapter Four

Following: The Magic of Palpation 129

Chapter Five
Holding: Creating a Safe Haven for the Patient and Family

Chapter Six
Moving Beyond Obstacles with Clarity and Purpose

Chapter Seven
Reflective Practice: The Means by Which Learning Becomes Permanent

Epilogue: A Return to Palpation

Foreword

The most unsettling experience I have had as a clinician was the day that one of my hospitalized patients took her life. To this day, the memory lingers.

The patient was a gentle, extraordinarily sensitive older woman who looked like a grandmother any of us would want to have. Her mother had died years earlier. She had no siblings and no children of her own, but she was the primary caregiver for her elderly father. While she spoke of wanting to die, the one concern that seemed to keep her from suicide was the need to care for her father.

At a time when the staff noted that she was feeling less depressed, she asked for a weekend pass to return home to visit her father and to see whether he was being well cared for in her absence. The pass was granted. On Sunday evening she returned to the hospital as planned. That evening she overdosed on hidden medications and died.

A root cause analysis exposed many factors contributing to her death. While policies and practices of the hospital were changed to safeguard patient safety going forward, there is no way to describe the effect her death had on the staff. I hope that no reader of this book will ever have a similar experience.

As unnerving as it was, however, it awakened in us a new awareness of our undeniable obligation to see beyond immediate appearances and to be sensitive to our patients' deepest needs. The book you hold in your hand will help us do that. Mary Koloroutis and Michael Trout have authored an inspirational and practical guide that shows us how to be present with our patients, to know their needs, and to see them as people.

Do you believe that the way in which you are present with your patients has an effect on their mental, emotional, spiritual, and even physical healing? Mary and Michael do. They contend that when we are truly present in the care of our patients, we're involved in what they and others have termed the *therapeutic relationship*. With the therapeutic relationship comes the probability of a more comprehensive and accelerated experience of healing. Without it, the human aspects of care are diminished, and healing may be diminished along with it.

As you read, ponder, question, and then integrate their insights into your daily work, you will discover or rediscover how amazingly practical this idea of the therapeutic relationship can be. At times, some of us have talked about this relationship as though it is mysterious and fleeting—as though it sometimes either happens or fails to happen through something other than our own thoughts and actions. But Mary and Michael have tied the therapeutic relationship to actions that can be easily understood and practiced with dedication. There is no mystery here. There is theory here, there is grounding in centuries of literature, there is reflection, and there are, perhaps most importantly, practical tools that every clinician in every discipline can use with every patient every time.

In *See Me as a Person*, the authors describe the three dynamics of the therapeutic relationship: the need to *wonder*, to *follow*, and to *hold*. These are unfamiliar terms for those of us accustomed to the more traditional language of medicine.

What does it mean to wonder, follow, and hold? Suffice it to say that a mind open to wonder is one ready to learn about, and even be surprised by, the person before you. To follow calls for an attuned ear, mind, and heart. To hold the patient and his or her family is to devote yourself to creating a safe haven for them. Among so many other things, it means that you watch over them to ensure that they don't have to contend with procedures for which they have not been adequately prepared or be subject to the use of unflattering labeling by your peers. If these thoughts are intriguing, you will relish this book.

This book is timely for three reasons. First, because many clinicians feel that it is no longer possible to work at a pace and with the attentiveness that patients need. The authors acknowledge the reality of the seemingly insurmountable obstacles caregivers face to being in authentic, unhurried relationships with patients, and they offer concrete suggestions on how to re-center ourselves and perhaps partner with others in order to preserve the integrity of patient-clinician relationships.

Secondly, the business side of health care is now front-and-center in the minds of many. Efficiency, bottom-line accountability, and measurable outcomes have entered our vocabulary and changed the way care is offered. Most would agree that the quality of patient care continues to improve. However, it is also true that in the process of change we have, at times, overlooked the key role that human relationships play in the healing process. Here again Mary and Michael have singular insights and suggestions on ways to make the human side of health care visible and actionable while also preserving and advancing its technical side. They emphasize that it is the balance of the human and technical sides of health care that makes optimal healing possible.

Thirdly, we live at a time when we refer to patients as customers. To think of them in this way has been helpful insofar as their satisfaction is uppermost in our minds as we work to make health care environments more welcoming and hospitable. However, patients differ from other kinds of customers in significant ways. In other milieus customers are in a position of control as they seek particular products or services. Patients, however, are largely dependent and uniquely vulnerable. They are frequently reluctant consumers of health care services and may be experiencing one of the worst times in their lives. Under these conditions, the authors propose, good customer service is not nearly enough. What is needed is knowledgeable and authentic clinicians who can meet people where they are, understand the magnitude and meaning of their illness to them, and help guide them toward recovery and healing.

While this book is needed and timely, do not expect a fast read. For instance the authors contend that the therapeutic relationship is like no other: clinicians do whatever is necessary to foster healing and expect literally nothing in return. Do you agree? They write that a "therapeutic relationship is not about 'being nice' or adhering to prescribed or scripted communications. Neither is a therapeutic relationship dependent upon the clinician's personality. It is knowledge-based and grounded in human caring science, research, and accumulated clinical wisdom." Again, do you agree? Or do these ideas stir discomfort in you?

Mary and Michael have a gift. They phrase their insights in a manner that is sometimes provocative. As I read through the text for the first time I wished they had been in the room with me so I could have questioned their thought process. Now, I am glad they were not. They made me think in fresh ways. I suspect you will find that the same is true for you. Consider these few thoughts among dozens that I could have chosen:

> *It takes no small measure of arrogance to think that one knows almost anything about a human being with whom he or she has not yet spent any time in relationship.*
>
> *Just as it would never be thought acceptable that a clinician would fail to be technically proficient, it can never be thought acceptable that a clinician be permitted to lack relational proficiency.*

If the patient has identified a family member as essential to his recovery, the family member becomes a member of the care team, not a visitor.

In a clinical setting, authentic human connection cannot be mandated. It can, however, be a clearly articulated expectation, a shared purpose, a goal, and a standard.

When clinicians show both compassion and empathy, a human connection of mutual vulnerability and intimacy creates a bond that may last no more than a moment, but that may heal wounds that have been carried for a lifetime.

You will find similarly provocative (and sometimes heart-rending) statements on almost every page.

See Me as a Person can be read in a few sittings, but that would be unfortunate. It deserves to be studied. In fact, its greatest value will be found when studied as a team. Whether physicians or nurses, administrators or managers, whether we work at the bedside or behind the scenes in supportive roles, Mary and Michael have shown us what it is necessary to do if we are to continually improve patient care. To them we are indebted.

During the extensive root cause analysis that followed the death of my patient, it was discovered that only one clinician, an art therapist, genuinely understood the patient's way of thinking during that regrettable weekend. Once my patient could see with her own eyes that her father was cared for, she could do what she had planned to do. Reflecting on those years as a young clinician, I wish I had read *See Me as a Person*. No, I wish that we as a team had studied it.

Martin C. Helldorfer

May 6, 2012

Co-author of *Healing with Heart: Inspirations for Health Care Professionals* and *Healthy Ways to Work in Health Care: A Self Care Guide.*

Preface

Whether you're a physician, nurse, technician, or therapist—it doesn't matter. I am your patient.

I'm lying in a hospital bed. It is 1993, and I am 18 years old—still a kid, really. But as you walk into my hospital room, you can't be quite sure I'm even human, much less a young guy. That patient in front of you—that would be *me*—only really looks human from the neck down. My arms are black and blue with bruises. There is road rash down my sides and more across my back. There is a J tube poking out from my belly. My legs are in traction and there are half a dozen pins protruding from each leg. These pins are in your care. Three times per day they are to be cleaned—an action which feels to me like a cigarette being crushed out on my skin.

It's lucky for me that you're such a steady person (though I don't really know that yet), because it's about to get a lot worse. As you look at my throat and make your way up to the top of my head, this is where it really gets ugly.

At the base of my throat is the tracheostomy. "Chipmunk cheeks" are nothing new to you; they're common to patients with facial injuries. You've also seen plenty of bandaged eyes from ophthalmologic surgeries, along with lots of staples and stitches. But if you add them all up, I don't look very much like a person. There is a four-inch flap of skin torn from across my chin. My lips are swollen, dry, and bleeding. My jaws are wired, and nearly all of my teeth are broken. My cheeks are scraped raw and peppered with scabs. Both of my eyes have been sewn shut and have been covered with thin metal trays attached by a wide strip of white medical tape and dressings. I am blind, but I don't know it yet.

I can barely think a lot of the time, but still I manage to worry that you'll see me as a monster or that you'll be so overcome with grief that you'll just want to do what you need to do and get out. I'm like that; I think about what other people might be experiencing. But you just keep your focus on me—on a *me* that is so much more than this horribly battered body. I don't know how you do that, and it's weird because even though I can't see you, I can feel that you're looking at me the way I'd want to be looked at right now. I can sense your compassion, your close attention to so many things about me all at the same time.

My parents are huddled in a corner trying to hold onto some sense of normalcy, but there's no escaping the fact that nothing will ever be the same again. My mother manages to speak. "Marcus. That's his name," she tells you, knowing that you already know, but not knowing where to begin. And then both of my parents tell you more so that you'll have a better sense of who Marcus the person really is—who they desperately need to believe I still am, despite what happened. You clearly welcome the information; even in my half-sleep, I can hear you settle in and make the smallest sounds in answer to the details of the story of who I am and what happened to me. It's clear that your heart is with this couple: middle-aged, salt of the earth parents who love their child. They're living through every parent's worst nightmare: a child changed forever simply because he found himself in the path of a drunk driver. You promise, you say, to help in any way you can. Your eyes, they will tell me later, show them the truth of your commitment to all of us.

Hours later, you hear the quiet conversation of a group of half a dozen young men gathering outside the half-open door of my room. You wonder if this is too many visitors at once. Is Marcus stable enough for such a large group of visitors? So you ask me, "Marcus, a bunch of guys are here to see you. Do you want them to come in?"

"Yes!" I scrawl across the yellow legal tablet that currently acts as my voice. The letters come so quickly, and with such certainty, that it takes you by surprise. While I have been nearly motionless, when I hear my friends and loved ones, I come alive. It's a tender moment as they huddle around my bed, each lightly laying a hand on me. It is, perhaps, not quite like anything you've witnessed before, this outpouring of support and compassion for one so young by his peers. This, you realize, is what will heal me emotionally and mentally, and you commit to doing what you can to safeguard these visits for me in the face of any objections you might meet from people on the floor.

While my buddies are there, my parents walk down to the waiting room. It's almost your break time, and you're concerned about them. They are always here. Always. My mother rarely leaves my bedside. "Can I take you down to the cafeteria for a cup of coffee?" you ask them. They both look up surprised. "I'm on break for the next 15 minutes and Marcus seems in really good hands with his friends," you say, offering them an encouraging smile.

Over a cup of coffee you ask more about me, and my parents are eager to share: former high school football player, goes by "Marc" to his friends, freshman at Missouri State, involved in church, big music fan, big sports fan, with more friends than they can count. They tell you how within 24 hours of the crash, more than 50 of my friends arrived from all over the state, and they aren't done filing in yet.

As the three of you talk, you learn that I am angry. At the drunk driver? At the prospect of never having any semblance of a normal life again? Well, yeah, but they know that my more immediate anger is aimed at the doctors and nurses who continually hurt me. You wonder about that for a moment, but it's not long before you're seeing it through my eyes. Every time a health care person comes into my room, they cause me pain. Pin care, dressing changes, alcohol swabs. My parents tell you I'm in such a fragile state that just barely bumping my bed sets off explosions of pain. You make a mental note that if I express anger toward you, you won't take it personally. I may say that I hate you for inflicting pain, and in that moment, I probably do. So you'll remember to allow time for the pain to subside. You'll give me time to adjust. You won't judge me or yourself in that moment.

When you return to the floor my friends are just leaving. Some are smiling, some are teary. "Everything go okay?" you ask. "Yeah, he gave us the finger," one says, tears mixed with smiles. "He's still in there," he says. Indeed, I am.

I am your patient. And I am a person with family, friends, faith, hopes, longings, and even (believe it or not) plans for the future. Everything you do or say that helps me feel seen as a person moves me one step closer to healing. Every time you help my family, you help me. Every time you hold my hand, I'm comforted. Every time you're in my room—because I know that you see me for who I really am—I feel safe.

I feel safe when you show me that you know what's important to my healing. When you make extra time for me to be with my friends and family—those people I've told you are so important to me—I feel safe again, and I begin to heal.

I feel safe when you respect my need for all of the things that help me feel more secure right now. You never give me grief for being a 250 lb. man with a stuffed animal tucked under my chin. You let me keep my music on because we've talked about how important it is to me. You ask me how my team did in the game I was listening to earlier, because the results have meaning for me, and that seems to matter to you.

I feel safe when you take care of my parents. You know that I worry about them all the time. I understand their loss more than anyone else does, and yet I'm powerless to do anything for them. When you do for me the things I'd do for myself if I could, I feel like you've got my back.

When I am released from the hospital after my first 46-day stay, it's Thanksgiving Day. The hospital is operating with a skeleton crew, and you, my favorite nurse, are home with your family. While I'm happy to be going home, I'm bummed that you're not there. After I'm all packed up and being wheeled down the hall, suddenly there you are, a gentle hand on my shoulder, and your familiar voice saying, "Nobody's sending my kid home but me."

I know that not all of your patients are as bad off as I am, but I also know that you're just as caring and attentive with them as you are with me. It's so obviously a part of you to give compassionate, competent care that it's not just the things you do that make a difference for me, it's the way you *are*. I don't know how you got this way, but I now know how other clinicians can learn to be more like you. The readers of this book are getting the chance to learn the elements of what you did with me and even to experience the essence of who you were with me. As a patient, I want every caregiver in every discipline to be at least a little like you.

And to that end, I'd like it very much if every caregiver read this book; heck, I'd kind of like them to memorize it.

See Me as a Person is a book about three practices that every caregiver can learn and apply no matter what his or her discipline. The practices are very straightforward and easy to understand, and in my opinion, they're essential. But I also know they're not always easy to do. They require that you be fully present and engaged, relating human-to-human with your patients. That's no small thing, but it also happens to be one of the things that helps your patients feel safe no matter how far they are, or will ever be, from full recovery.

Clearly my broken body was repaired through the remarkable technical competence of countless surgeons and other technically skilled clinicians. There is no question that my mind and my spirit were healed by the unshakable love of my family, my friends, and my faith. And there is also no question that when you cared about me as a person, I felt more able to let that love in. People ask me sometimes whether I'd rather have a super-competent caregiver or a kind and caring one. In truth, I always choose competence, but I'm also always irritated by the question. It makes no sense to me that this is a choice that a patient should ever be forced to make. Technical competence isn't optional; neither is kindness or genuine caring.

As a former patient, as someone who will probably be a patient again, as someone who will likely be a dear friend or family member of someone who will one day be in your care, and as a member of the human family, I'm grateful to every reader of this book. As you take steps to become an even more caring, compassionate caregiver, you hone the gift you've chosen to give to the world. I, for one, am grateful.

Marcus Engel

April 11, 2012
Author of *The Other End of the Stethoscope:*
33 Insights for Excellent Patient Care and *I'm Here:*
Compassionate Communication in Patient Care.

Acknowledgements

We thank the many nurses, physicians, therapists, and patients and families who have inspired us in this work through their stories, achievements, and struggles. We respect and appreciate all of you who bring care and compassion to life every day in this complex and confounding health care world of ours.

We are so very grateful and indebted to Rebecca Smith, our developmental editor, colleague, and collaborator in the writing of this book. Rebecca helped us integrate our individual voices and perspectives without relinquishing the gift of our unique contributions. She tirelessly helped us navigate the tough times and come out with something better than we ever could have without her grace, humor, skill, creativity, and absolute unrelenting commitment to excellence. Rebecca's purpose is to "beautify," and we appreciate all of the ways she helped us beautify the written word.

We appreciate all of the support and encouragement we received from the Creative Health Care Management team who tirelessly reviewed and edited the manuscript and supported its development in so many ways. We appreciate the thoughtful, meticulous editing work of Cathy Perrizo and Marty Lewis-Hunstiger as well as the invaluable fact checking of Rachel Haukkala. We are particularly grateful to Chris Bjork for his leadership and management of the publishing process including that special skill for keeping us on track with those ever-so-important timelines.

A special thank you to Jay Monroe for the creative and thoughtful design work which helps to bring this book to life.

Finally, we are grateful to all of our colleagues who believe in the work of human caring and the imperative for us to create more humane and compassionate health care services.

Mary Koloroutis and Michael Trout

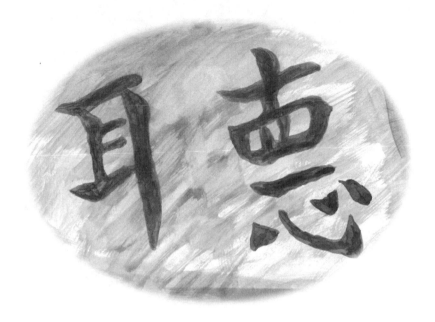

A piece of art which included this Chinese character was given to Michael by one of his patients. Its literal translation is, simply, "listen."

As she presented it to him, she told him that what it means to her is this:

You see me . . .

You listen to me . . .

You give me your undivided attention.

These words have inspired every word of this work.

Introduction

It was one of those spring days that is, in and of itself, an inspiration. Roger Ebert was in town, and we were joining many other film buffs for a three-day festival to view his picks for first-rate but unheralded movies. We went for a long walk between films, and that's where the idea for this book was born.

Mary had written and taught for years about Relationship-Based Care, the notion that health care could be markedly improved by attending to the connection between the clinician and patient, and that organizations can transform their cultures to surround, support, and make time for that connection.

Michael had written and taught for years about the nuances of the infant-parent relationship, that often-taken-for-granted and sometimes elusive attachment between baby and parent upon which much of the baby's development (sense of self, sense of self-with-others, capacity to trust) depends.

As a nurse, Mary knew a great deal about the practicalities of health care, and the enormous challenges faced by caregivers (particularly those in hospitals) who are trying to carve out time to connect with their patients, often with limited success.

As a counselor in private practice, Michael knew some things about the processes by which humans connect with each other both in therapy and in real life.

Both of us understood that the efficacy of care—and perhaps just as importantly, the patient's experience of care—depends heavily on authentic human connection. Patients in Michael's practice didn't get better because he was clever or used good tactics or strategies. They got better when they experienced his empathy, his earnest efforts to understand them by hearing their stories, and when they re-experienced old hurts in this new relationship with someone who, this time around, wouldn't hurt them.

Both of us understood that the efficacy of care—and perhaps just as importantly, the patient's experience of care—depends heavily on authentic human connection.

Stirred by portrayals of anger and violence in some of the films we'd seen at the festival, we began exchanging stories about patients' anger and soon realized that we shared a perspective: anger was not "bad behavior"; anger was meaningful, a signal that the angry person was terrified and needed to sound the alarm that he was feeling powerless and without other more rational resources. Could the same be true about other difficult patient behaviors or patient/family behaviors: resistance to procedures, excessive dependence, or demandingness, for example? Could many of these behaviors, which so complicate the already difficult day of many clinicians, be dealt with more easily if they were understood and responded to as actual communications, and could such an approach save time in the long run?

Still reveling in the early spring sun and kicking leaves left over from the previous fall, we stepped into the most uplifting possibility of all: Could it be that health care providers already have knowledge and skills which, if used with intention, could dramatically increase the speed of recovery, improve the patient's experience in the hospital, calm the units, and increase the caregiver's sense of meaning and purpose?

A model became apparent to us for describing exactly what comprises the experience of authentic human connection. We thought we could describe what happens between patient and caregiver in terms that would have immediate meaning and applicability to clinicians in any health care discipline. We saw the possibility for a book that presented three highly effective therapeutic practices and actually helped clinicians from all disciplines understand how to integrate them into their own daily practice.

We have observed that many books presuming to be how-to books actually end up being why-to books. They make the case for a *way of being* or a *way of doing,* but they don't actually tell you how to do anything. A book about relationships is an especially thorny endeavor from this perspective. Relationships are based on authenticity, so how can it be that anyone could write a book that "taught" people how to be in authentic relationship with each other? As we talked, three practices emerged fairly quickly and came to the forefront. We decided that these three practices not only could be taught, but that they were already happening in satisfying patient experiences. We tested them in conversations with peers and then with groups in our workshops, and we saw that people were responding. It was clear that they were hungry for practical and accessible ways to be authentically present with the people they cared for, even as they also felt discouraged by the complexities and pressures of the health care world.

We offer to you, herein, a clear, practical encapsulation of the elements of human connection as they are expressed in the health care setting. We bring to you three therapeutic practices that we call *wondering, following,* and *holding.* They are practices which create authentic connection when clinicians are present and attuned to their patients.

We first explore our natural capacity to attune and how it can help us to be more present and accessible to the people in our care. Within that overall mindset of attunement, we hope that you will find *wondering* about your patients to be as uplifting, both for you and for the patient, as we propose it can be. We will suggest what it means to *follow* your patient, and the implications of such an uncommon (but we think, intuitive) behavior for getting an accurate health history, a true response to daily inquiries, or an understanding of why this patient's brother is so burdensome to the staff or why the patient presses the call button so often. We will consider with you what it is like to *hold* a patient, in every sense of the word, and what it is like for the patient and family to truly feel *held* in our care.

Paradoxically, although it's likely that you'll learn many new things in this book, it's far from true that this book will burden you with more things to remember. Wondering, following, and holding actually represent a return to a level of deep human connection that is likely written quite strongly into your professional "muscle memory" already. It's likely that in the time it takes for you to read this book, its concepts will begin to integrate themselves into your work and even into your personal life. Ultimately, this is a book about relationships, so it seems more than conceivable that you'll feel the truth of it in your bones. You may even recognize it as a return to your own deepest truth. Perhaps it represents a new way for you to understand that thing you could never quite put your finger on, that describes why you went into health care in the first place.

We think you'll discover that you already practice wondering, following, and holding in your most satisfying patient encounters. But sometimes, unless those peak experiences are deconstructed for us, we're not entirely certain of

> *Although it's likely that you'll learn many new things in this book, it's far from true that this book will burden you with more things to remember.*

what comprises them. We may even refer to them as "magic moments," placing them well outside the realm of the replicable. We may look at the work of a colleague and determine that she just "has it," . . . and that, perhaps, we don't.

But you do have it. In your best moments you're doing all or most of these four things:

1. You're being fully present with "this person right now," attuning to who he or she is as a human being.

2. You're suspending your conclusions as you ask questions and listen carefully for answers that make wonder an integral part of the relationships you build.

3. You're following the cues you're getting from the person in front of you, venturing into new inquiries based directly on both the verbal and nonverbal answers you're receiving.

4. You're metaphorically (and sometimes literally) holding the person in a way that demonstrates that you will do what it takes to safeguard the other from physical, mental, and emotional harm no matter what might threaten to interfere with your connection.

It sounds familiar, doesn't it? If you are a clinician within any discipline in the world of health care, we're certain that you've experienced every one of these four things.

Authentic Connection and Patient Satisfaction

Michael offers this remembrance of an experience of authentic connection that has stayed with him for more than half a lifetime:

Ruby

I vividly remember what it was like to walk into the old, downtown diner in Traverse City, Michigan, 35 years ago. I never knew the waitress's name, though I call her "Ruby" in my mind; somehow that appellation captures her warmth, her age (advanced), and her no-nonsense sweetness.

She never wrote anything down. She just listened with such care that she could easily walk back to the cook's window and repeat the order perfectly. This was only the first sign of her astounding efficiency. Every move she made had the mark of a pro. It didn't stress her a bit that she was often in charge of the whole joint on her own, such was her professionalism, her dignity, her speed, her capacity to take care of business with zero wasted effort. How was she able to simultaneously carry on the way she did with her customers and get everything to every table without missing a beat?

If you had been there more than twice she knew your name and she used it to address you. If you didn't eat your carrots she would needle you until you did (or until you erupted with such laughter that you could scarcely eat anything). She would remember that you liked your hash browns crispy and would sometimes take the plate back to have the cook make it right before you could even think to complain. When she asked about how the breakfast suited you, she asked in such a way that you imagined she was really looking out for your satisfaction, your health, your nurturance.

Ruby may have honed her talents on the discharged or day-pass patients from the huge mental hospital nearby. She fussed over them in a way that likely contributed to their success in the outside world. However she came by her abilities, Ruby was a professional, and no program or system was ever needed to motivate her to be interested in "the customer experience." I suspect there was never an argument in her mind about whether she had time to look after her relationships with her customers. Ruby was not there to serve up meals; she was there to feed her people.

Her incredible efficiency allowed her to do exactly that in less time than it would take many waitresses to stumble through a shift while barely noticing their customers as individual people at all. The well-done burger with no pickles never went to "table four"; it went to Jack.

Unbeknownst to Ruby, she had a profound impact on how I would practice psychotherapy for the next several decades. She listened. She watched out for people. Her interest in people was sincere and unshakeable. She was infinitely kind, and she brought an authentic, well-timed playfulness that lifted people. In my best moments, I can only hope that I connect with the true purpose of my work and the people in my care as Ruby did.

Some institutions, despairing of the possibility of clinicians ever being able to build authentic relationships with patients, will set out to mimic the rudiments of relatedness. If we say the words that people might say if they were in a relationship, maybe we can get away with not actually having one.

Because you are holding this book in your capable and curious hands, we suspect that you might be thinking a little more deeply about patient satisfaction. We suspect you might be wondering how to build a culture that makes possible the sort of patient experience that shows up in elevated HCAHPS scores.

We are entering a time in health care which is challenging for many reasons, not the least of which is that attending to the patient experience now has dollars attached to it. This will be a headache for some and an opportunity for others. How we interpret patient satisfaction and how we go about the job of improving our HCAHPS scores will reflect the values and beliefs of the cultures in which we practice.

Standardizing a culture of therapeutic relationships is tough. We will stumble, but if we remember why we're interested in the patient experience, we may be able to improve it. At Carolinas HealthCare System, employees were trained to use a variety of "tactics," including listening to patients for two minutes without interruption and regularly using expressions such as, "I want to make sure I understood you correctly" (Bush, 2011, p. 24). Admittedly, this could come out all wrong, with staff using the tactic but forgetting the actual experience of relating. On the other hand, it could be brilliant. If staff actually committed to the spirit as well as the letter of the tactic, they could find themselves becoming genuinely interested in the patient during that sacred two minutes of uninterrupted listening. Any follow-up questions might become meaningful to the clinician who really does become invested in whether or not she has understood correctly.

The Chief Patient Experience Officer at the Cleveland Clinic has noted that patients perceive their doctor to have spent much more time in the room with them if the doctor happens to have been sitting down during the exchange (Bush, 2011). So do we standardize sitting down as a key strategy for improving patient satisfaction? It might work quite well if we did. Mandating something as innocuous yet effective as sitting is not likely to interfere with the clinician's authenticity; in fact it could serve as a practical cue for becoming more attuned and present.

Scripting, however, is another matter.

"Hi, my name is Sandy, and I'll be your waitress this evening." Why is it that this scripted introduction—now in wide use in restaurants around the country, evidently because someone thought it would be an effective way to upgrade the customer experience—comes off as so empty?

Perhaps it's because it is empty. Can you imagine Ruby, the magnificently attuned server in Michael's memory, saying exactly the same thing to each unique person she encountered?

The Chief Medical Officer at Parkview Health System in Fort Wayne, Indiana has concluded that scripting will not get the job done and that improvements due to scripting are not sustainable (Bush, 2011). He teaches instead the value of curiosity as one of the core elements in creating a therapeutic relationship. This is the direction of our thinking as well. The therapeutic practices of wondering, following, and holding take us out of the world of scripting and give us a framework, principles, and language to authentically engage with this person, right now.

Wendy Austin, nursing professor and research chair at the Dossetor Health Ethics Center at the University of Alberta, writes that corporate and commercial values undermine nursing as a moral practice, and she challenges the "paradigm shift in which healthcare environments are viewed as marketplaces rather than moral communities" (p. 158). She proposes that the "corporate push" toward standardization and predictability means that care becomes a commodity rather than a moral action built on a sacred trust. This paradigm, Austin argues, is focused on "customer loyalty" (keeping and building business) rather than patient healing, and is thus a self-serving paradigm which interferes with building an authentic therapeutic relationship (p. 160).

We're a sophisticated society. There are customer service initiatives in action everywhere, and we can feel the difference between what's sincere and what's not. It's nice that a bank has great customer service. We love that when we walk into our bank someone greets us and helps us to get into the right line or to have a seat with the assurance that our banker is being notified of our arrival. There is no question that these practices have as their primary aim helping the customer feel oriented and well-taken care of, and that they help customers feel as though the bank is not in the business of ignoring them or wasting their time.

But it's what happens next that determines whether these systems will leave us feeling held or dropped by those who appear to be taking such good care of us. If the next person who speaks to us uses the exact same greeting as the first person did, the sincerity of both greetings is suddenly in question. We perceive at that point that we're being "handled." Rather than allow ourselves to be fooled into thinking that anybody is interested in building a relationship with us, we see that they're doing only what they've been mandated by policy to do. If one person tells us to have an "outstanding" day we may think it a little extreme, though possibly charming in its oddity. But if we hear it twice in three minutes, it feels more like an insult to our intelligence than a sincere wish for our happiness. We know the difference between people who are trying to build authentic relationships with us and people who have said nice things to us because they are directed to do so.

We know the difference between people who are trying to build authentic relationships with us and people who have said nice things to us because they are directed to do so.

This is, however, just a bank. Most of the people walking into a bank are not sick or injured, while in a health care setting nearly everyone is vulnerable due to illness, injury, or deep concern for the well-being of a loved one. We have observed that people's sensitivity to insincerity and disconnection gets stronger when they're vulnerable. Patients and families are hyper-alert. They're the reason that this Maya Angelou quote gets so much play: "I've learned that people will forget what you said, people will forget what you did, but people will never forget how you made them feel." We repeat it often, not just because it describes the truth of our past experience, but because it has the power to inform everything we do for our patients and their families from here on out. When we create a practice built on tactics, techniques, and prescribed behaviors we risk limiting the ability of clinicians to connect as human beings, making them feel vigilant about what to say rather than *how to be* with their patients.

The ultra-efficient, customer-centered approach that the bank has for making sure that customers are greeted, oriented, and shepherded through their visits is essential to customer satisfaction, yet it is in no way a substitute for authentic, responsive relationships. Efficient systems are what make time for authentic relationships to happen. Good systems and good relationships are interdependent.

Why Human Connection is as Essential for Clinicians as it is for Patients and their Families

What do you suppose ever became of Ruby? Do you suppose she quit, certain that she could do better financially or perhaps find work a little closer to home? Do you suppose—well, can you even fathom the possibility—that she burned out?

Given what you know about how much of herself Ruby put into her work and how much nourishment she received from the people she so attentively fed, it seems likely that Ruby found a way of being in her work that was 100% sustainable. She fed others (literally and metaphorically) and she allowed herself to be in relationship with those she fed in a way that kept her energized. It could be said that she found meaning in her work, but it's far more accurate to say that she put meaning into her work through her decision to be in authentic, spontaneous relationship, if only for a short time, with everyone who came into "her" restaurant.

There is no question that some of Ruby's customers were more challenging than others. Some came in with chips on their shoulders and perhaps even with grudges against waitresses and restaurants in particular. Others found fault with anything she brought them, but Ruby knew that her job was to take care of people, and she also knew that people with chips on their shoulders and those who complained about everything were starved for something. She may or may not have been able to put her finger on the idea that what these people were starved for was human connection, but since that's what she so skillfully administered in these instances, she obviously knew it.

There are boundaries within the therapeutic relationship that might lead us to starve ourselves as caregivers from the very thing that keeps us going: "Don't get too involved with any one patient." . . . "Let it go, and go on to the next person." . . . "There's only so much you can do."

All of these admonishments have merit and all are meant to protect the caregiver from pain, vulnerability, and even burnout and compassion fatigue, but if we take them too far and shut ourselves off from human connection with our patients, our empathy will shut down. Before too long, we'll find ourselves walking through our day more focused on getting to the end of it than we are on connecting with our patients, their families, or our team members. (A tool for reflection on therapeutic boundaries can be found in Appendix A on page 388.)

It's one of those things that Ruby knew, or perhaps that she just intuitively did. She connected, and from that continual movement toward connection she got what she herself needed in order to keep going: she got human connection.

The therapeutic relationship is defined by some as a completely unselfish relationship. The needs of the caregiver are not supposed to be met in the therapeutic relationship. But while we believe that this is a boundary that must continually be tended to and reflected upon, the caregiver, being human, also has a need for human connection.

It is too easy in our chaotic, time-constrained health care environments to substitute niceties for connection, and it is very difficult to understand the level to which you may be making this substitution yourself without some reflection on that subject. We invite you to ask yourself these questions:

- Do I ever use niceness to mask my true feelings? Is this sometimes necessary? Is this sometimes appropriate? What effect does it have on my relationships?

- How often, if ever, do I enter a patient's room or invite a patient in for an appointment before I'm mentally or emotionally ready to focus, listen, and connect?

- What do I "get" in my best patient encounters? How do I feel about "getting something" within the therapeutic relationship?

The aim of this book is not to shatter current conventions in health care. Indeed it does far more to refine them than it does to revolutionize them. We have discovered that there are subtleties in practice that merit close reflection, peer discussion, and, in some cases, an upgrade. As you'll see, reflection plays a very important role in this book. We are far less interested in telling anyone how to practice differently than we are in helping clinicians to look more closely at their practice and to make more conscious decisions about how they will show up in their relationships with the people in their care, as well as with their team members.

Who is This Book For?

This is a book for clinicians, decision makers, and all stakeholders in the world of health care who are inspired by the constant, challenging reminder that illness and injury are complicated and that while all of our technology is wondrous, it's not the totality of health care; it's just a part of it.

When we've written about relationships so far, it has been to point out the vital importance of establishing an authentic human connection between patients, patients' families, and the clinicians who care for them. But the truth is that those relationships happen most frequently and most easily when other relationships within health care settings are designed to support the clinician-patient relationship. We are not naïve about the time constraints and chaotic environments in which nearly all clinicians work. We know that most clinicians are not given (at least not in any recognizable way) ample time to spend with their patients. We also know that human connection can happen in a moment and that ample time is not a prerequisite for connection. We have experienced the transformative power of turning one's full attention, for even one brief moment, to another human being in order to receive without judgment his concerns, his worries, perhaps his new and terrifying experience of vulnerability that threatens to crush him. This is a book for people who are not afraid to remember how much we human beings need each other.

This is a book for people who are not afraid to remember how much we human beings need each other.

There are no disciplines within health care in which the human beings who come to us are not experiencing vulnerability. It's the nature of the beast; we help people who are hurting. It's reasonable, then, that we might want to distance ourselves from that hurt. If we keep busy we can distract ourselves from the pain of others. We're taught to keep an emotional distance from our patients, and it is true that if we were to bring a completely naked empathy to all of our encounters with all of our patients we risk drowning in their seemingly infinite sorrows. But we believe that there is a middle ground that has been lost. Technology has increased at a rate that has challenged us to keep a balance between the technical and human aspects of our care. When we lose the balance between the technical and human aspects of our care, our patients and their families suffer and so do we. The Schwartz Center for Compassionate Health Care (2012) has gathered and interpreted research on the value of compassionate connections between health care clinicians and patients and their families. According to the Schwartz Center research, effective patient-caregiver communication and relationships are associated with these measurable outcomes:

1. Enhanced patient satisfaction

2. Informed, shared decision making

3. Increased adherence to recommended treatments

4. Improved health outcomes

5. Reduced malpractice claims

While it certainly helps that we have credible research demonstrating the cause-and-effect connection between compassionate care and better clinical and business outcomes, research alone doesn't make change happen. Connection cannot be mandated, and it would be ridiculous to think that anyone can be chastened into creating authentic human connections with patients, families, and team members. Instead, authentic human connection must be demonstrated continually and courageously by those to whom it comes easily, and it must be actively, compassionately cultivated in those to whom it does not.

Therapeutic care requires that clinical professionals do these three things:

- Practice with competence, both technically and relationally.

- Establish authentic connections.

- Convey compassion, empathy, and an understanding of the meaning and magnitude of the patient's illness or injury to the patient and family.

Unless these things occur, people do not feel seen or safe, and their prospect for long-term healing may be compromised. We are thus called to create cultures of excellence that result in a focus on healing and wholeness through authentic human interactions at every level and in every relationship.

This book is first and foremost for individual clinicians who are willing to do what it takes to create authentic relationships with the people in their care. It is also for health care teams who recognize the importance of the therapeutic relationship and come together to assure that each clinician-patient relationship is supported and protected. And it's for health care leaders who have the moral obligation to build and sustain the organizational conditions in which humane and compassionate care can thrive.

We have chosen the word *clinician* as the term to refer to professional health care providers from many disciplines: physicians, nurses, physical therapists, social workers, chaplains, speech therapists, occupational therapists, case managers, psychologists and more.

Today we may call ourselves clinician, team member, or health care leader; tomorrow we may be calling ourselves patient.

This book is for all of us. Today we may call ourselves clinician, team member, or health care leader; tomorrow we may be calling ourselves patient.

Overview of Chapters

Chapter One—The Nature of the Therapeutic Relationship

This chapter looks at the difference between the instrumental and the relational aspects of health care. While instrumental (technical) proficiency is necessary for curing the body, tending to the relational aspects of care is necessary for comprehensive healing. This chapter introduces the conscious practice of being present through attuning to those in our care, along with the therapeutic practices of wondering, following, and holding in terms of daily words and actions that help us to focus on seeing our patients and their families as people. The therapeutic relationship is not a way to "be nice" but rather a way of relating that facilitates the patient's or family members' ability to cope with their circumstances, to understand the meaning of this episode of illness or injury in their lives, and to take ownership for their own healing and recovery.

Chapter Two—Presence through Attunement

Attunement is what happens when connection is made because each person experiences the other as present. It is through attuning to another that we begin to form a relationship with that person and to enter each other's world. Our experience becomes aligned. The capacity to attune to our patients and families is a prerequisite for therapeutic care. Although attunement is a conscious practice, it's not a task to be performed; it's an intentional use of the self and it is the container for the therapeutic practices of wondering, following, and holding.

Chapter Three—Wondering: Cultivating Curiosity for Efficient and Compassionate Practice

The therapeutic practice of wondering asks clinicians to cultivate a state of mind characterized by curiosity, openness, and acceptance. It's a joyful not-knowing and an intentional elimination of our own agenda. This chapter explores the myriad ways that wondering helps us to reach beyond what we think we already know, into a mindset of discovery that helps our patients to get the best possible care while energizing ourselves in the process.

Chapter Four—Following: The Magic of Palpation

The therapeutic practice of following guides clinicians toward a series of intentional acts that demonstrate devotion on the part of the clinician to being led and taught by the patient and family. This chapter explains the benefits of listening deeply to what our patients and their families are saying, as well as paying close attention to what they're not saying, so that we can customize our care in ways that help them to feel seen and safe and to heal more completely and more quickly.

Chapter Five—Holding: Creating a Safe Haven for the Patient and Family

The therapeutic practice of holding is a conscious decision to lift up, affirm, and dignify that which the patient or family member has taught us, resulting in intense focus on the patient or family member while treasuring both the information and the person. This chapter is an in-depth exploration of the very practical measures we can take to help our patients and their families feel that we as clinicians, and the health care organizations in which we work, are tending at all times to their physical safety, their emotional well-being, and the preservation of their dignity.

Chapter Six—Moving Beyond Obstacles with Clarity and Purpose

It is clear that the obstacles we face in our practice are real and at times quite daunting. The four obstacles to the therapeutic relationship most often identified by participants in our workshops are: 1) chaotic work environments; 2) time constraints; 3) patient and family anger; and 4) the clinician's judging mind. This chapter offers a way of thinking and practical strategies for moving beyond these obstacles to establish therapeutic relationships with every patient and family in our care.

Chapter Seven—Reflective Practice: The Means by Which Learning Becomes Permanent

This chapter explains the method by which reflection on our caregiving experiences makes us stronger clinicians as it helps us to transform the data and information of our experiences into lasting wisdom. A number of individual and group reflection techniques and formats are offered.

How to Get the Most from This Book

We want to take a moment to orient you to some of the features of this book so that you can more easily use its content for your own personal work as well as in group discussions and development activities. The distinct features of the book include its use of rich source material, personal stories, chapter summaries, reflection questions, and alternating gender-specific pronouns to maintain gender neutrality.

Rich Source Material

This book is based on a foundation of interdisciplinary literature and research. We draw from published findings in nursing, psychology, and medical journals as well as the worlds of business, management, leadership, communication, and philosophy. We also cite ideas from poetry and spiritual writings. Our work is informed by science and fed by truths that cross over into art, morality, and beyond. It's our hope that by providing rich source material we will be able to reach a diverse readership and speak to different facets within individual readers.

Personal Stories

Author Brenè Brown says that "stories are data with a soul" (Brown, 2010). They are ways to interpret the past and to be intentional about the future. They can help us to move beyond our simple cognitive thinking into accessing our emotional feelings about situations, which can then lead us to new insights and deepen our understanding.

We use a great deal of story in this book, and we want you to know that it's not without a voice over our shoulder saying "This is an anecdote. What legitimacy does it have? Just because it happened to one, is it universal?" We have chosen some stories that are universal, but just as often we have chosen stories that are merely instructive, illustrating—with realistic if not always universal examples—the practices this book is advocating. The stories are meant to deepen the reader's understanding of the concepts and to aid in your ability to integrate the material into your own practice more easily.

Many of our stories have come from participants in our workshops, with their kind permission. Our workshop participants include patients and their families as well as clinicians. Other stories come from our colleagues, from exemplars in the field, and from written surveys. We also draw on our own clinical practices for stories, though we take care to change details in order to protect individuals' privacy. There are also many stories that come from our own experiences as patients, as adult children of aging and dying parents, and as the parents of our young adult daughter who suffers with a chronic illness. In her journey, more than any other, we have learned about what health care looks like from "the other side of the door."

Chapter Summaries and Reflection Material

Each chapter ends with a Summary of Key Thoughts. These make for easy review of the chapters as well as quick references for readers who wish to return to specific chapters for more in-depth review. The Reflection section that ends each chapter provides material for ongoing reflection, encouraging the integration of the concepts presented in the chapter. As will be discussed and well supported later, reflection is a necessary part of learning any concept, particularly one that is meant to be integrated into our ongoing practice. We do not "own" any learning until we have reflected upon it and taken action to put it into practice.

Use of Pronouns for Gender Neutrality

Throughout this book we have attempted to maintain gender neutrality by referring to patients, family members, and clinicians, using a method of alternating masculine and feminine pronouns equally. We have chosen this method rather than using the sometimes cumbersome *he or she* or the grammatically not-yet-standard *they* when using a pronoun to refer to an individual in instances where the individual could be of either gender.

Our Invitation to You

We hope this book will validate the power of your work and help you to see each person in your care as a unique human being who deserves dignity, respect, and compassion. We hope that together we can push past the obstacles, the tasks, the time constraints, and all the other reasons why it is too hard to see each person and hold him intentionally in our care. Peter Block, in his book *The Answer to How is Yes* (2002), writes about the human tendency to give up on what truly matters, and in so doing, to sacrifice ourselves as well as those we serve. He says:

> *There is something in the persistent question How? that expresses each person's struggle to live a life of purpose [while] yielding to the daily demands of being practical. It is entirely possible to spend our days engaged in activities that work well for us and achieve our objectives and still wonder whether we are really making a difference in the world. My premise is that this culture and we as members of it, have yielded too easily to what is doable and practical. In the process we have sacrificed the pursuit of what is in our hearts. . . . We might put aside our wish for safety and instead view our life (and our practice) as a purpose-filled experiment whose intention is more for learning than for achieving and more for relationship than for power, speed, or efficiency. (pp. 1, 3)*

Block's words invite us to push past the obstacles and pursue what is most important and fulfilling for the people in our care and for ourselves. He asks us to say, "Yes." We invite you to as well.

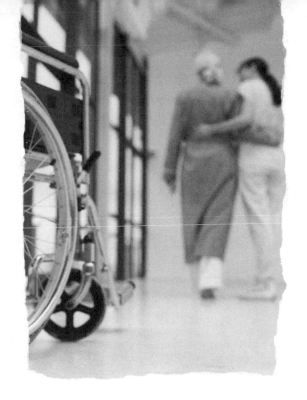

Chapter One

The Nature of the
Therapeutic Relationship

*Everyone who is born holds dual citizenship in the
kingdom of the well and in the kingdom of the sick.
Although we all prefer to use only the good passport,
sooner or later each of us is obliged, at least for a spell, to
identify ourselves as citizens of that other place.*

—Susan Sontag

Maria Bellchambers, who serves as Director of the Emergency Department at Laurel Regional Hospital in Maryland, shared with us this personal story from her early days in nursing (personal communication, June 26, 2011). In it she illustrates how she was taught to remain grounded and compassionate when people's behavior seemed to push her away.

The Cloak

They called the war in Ireland "the Troubles." It's funny how people put an acceptable name on an unacceptable situation.

In nursing school, the teachers were very clear that we were going to have to deal with the Troubles. We had classes where they would discuss what we were going to experience. Royal Victoria Hospital (opened by Queen Victoria in Belfast in 1873) would get its share of traumas, burns—everything but organ transplants.

The people involved in the Troubles were as varied as they were rancorous—the British Army, the Ulster Police, the Irish Republican Army (Catholic), the Ulster Freedom Fighters (Protestant), paramilitary splinter groups, and even politicians and clergy. And with that many factions all fighting each other in Belfast, we knew that we would see victims of violence and that some of those victims would very likely have tried their best to hurt people we loved.

The hospital was patrolled by army and police officers with machine guns. When I tell that to people they shudder sometimes, but we felt protected by their presence. We might be blown up walking down the street or riding on a bus, but the hospital was secured.

Royal Victoria Hospital was a Protestant hospital, so I knew that I would have patients who would curse at me because they would know by my name (Maria) that I was a Catholic. It was inevitable that they would abuse me verbally. The teachers knew that would happen so they prepared us.

They taught us about our sacred mission that came down from Florence Nightingale. She took herself into the most dire conditions during the Crimean War. She knew that the patients needed dignity and respect. Our teachers taught us that it was part of our mission that even though the patients may yell at us or curse at us, we won't react or take it as an affront to our personhood. We understood that we could never allow the patient to break through the cloak, as we called it—we wore capes in those days, which were a symbol of the dignity of our profession—with the ugliness they were trying to attach to us.

Our teachers told us, "Your dignity, your mission, your values ... that's what you bring to the bedside and don't allow anyone to take that away from you." They taught us that we would retain our souls and our mission if we'd not allow the ugliness to break through and touch us. If we reacted and allowed it to break through and allowed that sacredness to be violated, it would all be lost.

When we didn't react to their taunts and insults, it had an effect on the patients; if we didn't react they wouldn't continue, and the only thing that echoed was their own words.

Our school gave us the tools we needed by reminding us about our mission and where it came from. I use it to this day in the emergency department. Sometimes patients have been abused and don't know kindness. If you truly do center yourself, when they look into your eyes they will see kindness, and when you don't center yourself and you react, they see your fear or that you're judging them.

I teach that you center yourself, you get down, right in front of them, look them in the eye with all of that kindness and say,

"I want to take those handcuffs off but you have to work with me."

If you treat patients with kindness and dignity they see it. And they respond to it. I observed a couple of staff members step in when a fellow nurse was being too harsh with a patient. I could see that these staff members are proud of themselves, their practice, and their mission—proud that they can stay compassionate and committed no matter what.

The Purpose of the Therapeutic Relationship

The therapeutic relationship is like no other. In personal relationships an agreeable balance of give and take is often prized, but there is no such balance in the therapeutic relationship. In the therapeutic relationship the clinician offers care, touch, compassion, presence, and any other act or attitude that would foster healing, and expects nothing in return.

The word "therapeutic" comes from the Greek *therapeuein*, which means to minister to or attend to another. To minister means to give service, care, or aid; to attend to the needs, wants, or necessities of another being; to contribute to comfort or happiness.

In our world—one in which we may not experience widespread upsets like "the Troubles"—Maria Bellchambers' story may seem like an extreme example, but even today Maria reports that she still sees similar dynamics in her emergency room so many years later. It still takes grounding for us to remain compassionate when people's behavior is pushing us away. In theory no one argues against the need for care and dignity for all, but in the face of the ugliness that will sometimes appear in clinical settings we all need the preparation and support that it takes in order to stay therapeutic when people are not so easy to be with.

No matter who the patient is, the purpose of the therapeutic relationship remains the same: to connect with another *as a person* in order to facilitate his or her healing. To help us embody that purpose, this chapter will offer the research, theory, principles, and practices that explain and support the therapeutic relationship—a relationship that requires a masterful balance of both the instrumental and relational aspects of care (Benner, Sutphen, Leonard, & Day, 2010).

In health care, our varying disciplines and roles are built on distinct bodies of instrumental knowledge. Psychologists, physical therapists, physicians, nurses, and other clinicians are educated in distinctly different ways in order to prepare them to perform distinctly different clinical functions. However, the art and science of caring—the relational knowledge needed in order to minister to another—is a shared responsibility for clinicians across the entire spectrum of healing disciplines. Just as it would never be thought acceptable that a clinician would fail to be technically proficient, it can never be thought acceptable that a clinician be permitted to lack relational proficiency. It is a matter of both ethical and professional accountability for clinicians in every field of health care to relate therapeutically with every person in their care.

Just as it would never be thought acceptable that a clinician would fail to be technically proficient, it can never be thought acceptable that a clinician be permitted to lack relational proficiency.

In the best of care, in every clinical discipline, there is an elegant balance of the relational and instrumental aspects of care. It's possible for all medical interventions to be carried out within the relational context, but too often the relational gets pushed aside in the name of efficiency. This is ironic, as it is often the lack of relational proficiency that causes clinicians to have to spend additional time repeating themselves, reorienting people, or calming people down. Including the relational aspect of care can be as simple as asking the patient if he or she is ready for what's coming next.

When the relational aspects of care are attended to, people tend to feel less often as though things are being done to them. Instead people feel as though they and their caregivers are working together toward their healing. It's important to note also that the relational aspects of care comprise the sum total of the care that we can provide for the patient's family. Since no medical interventions are part of the family's care, the value of the relational aspects of our care for them is inestimable. We submit that every medical intervention can be done in a way that preserves and supports the clinician-patient relationship. When the instrumental and relational aspects of care are integrated in a masterful balance, healing takes place whether or not cure is possible.

Still, all too often we perpetuate the separation of human caring and connection (essential for healing) from the technical-scientific nature of our practice (essential for curing) when we see either as superior to the other. When this happens we ignore the fact that relational and technical knowledge are intrinsically interconnected in clinical work. And we propose that the more technically complex our health care environments get, the more important the relational aspects of care become. As illustrated in Figure 1.1 on the following page, when caring for the whole person in a way that puts her in the best position for both curing and healing we will consistently integrate both the instrumental and the relational aspects of our work.

There's a necessary symmetry to the work of curing and healing. The instrumental and relational aspects of our practice call on us to use knowledge and skills that are as distinct as they are complementary.

FIGURE 1.1: Balancing Relational and Instrumental Care

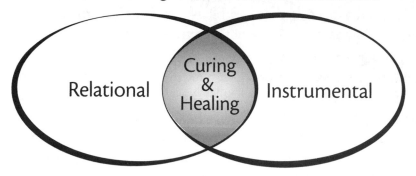

The therapeutic relationship differs significantly from social or collegial relationships in which the needs of both parties are of mutual concern. In the therapeutic relationship the needs of the person receiving care are of overriding concern, and the needs of the clinician are intentionally attended to elsewhere. In the therapeutic relationship, through the intentional use of self, caregivers cultivate emotional safety for their patients and, when applicable, to the patients' loved ones. In these relationships, clinicians focus on three key capacities in their patients:

- The clinician facilitates the person's ability to cope with the circumstances she is facing.

- The clinician facilitates the person's ability to understand the meaning of the episode of illness or injury in her life.

- The clinician nurtures the person's desire to take ownership for her own healing, and therefore, to take the best possible actions for immediate and ongoing recovery and/or management of her disease process.

As our recap of these three capacities suggests, the purpose of the therapeutic relationship is to promote, guide, and support the healing of another person through knowledgeable and authentic connection. Within the world of health care, the act of therapeutic connection is not owned by practitioners of any one discipline. The responsibility to offer care to another human being is something we all share. This striving to create connection in the service of care gives us a common purpose that unites us as health care professionals.

What the Therapeutic Relationship Is, and What It Is Not

As we think about what the therapeutic relationship is, it is also important to be cognizant that the therapeutic relationship is not about "being nice" or adhering to prescribed or scripted communications or action. The therapeutic relationship is not dependent upon the clinician's personality. The therapeutic relationship is built on authentic words and actions. It is knowledge-based and grounded in human caring science, research, and accumulated clinical wisdom.

In a clinical setting, authentic human connection cannot be mandated. It can, however, be a clearly articulated expectation, a shared purpose, a goal, and a standard. In our work with health care professionals we sometimes hear people voice the opinion that you either have "the caring gene" or you don't— that it is something innate rather than something that can be learned and developed as part of our professional competency. We propose that while it may be true that caring is a more natural capacity for some than for others (just as some have more natural technical capacity) we don't get a pass in developing our relational skills simply because it isn't easy for

> In a clinical setting, authentic human connection cannot be mandated. It can, however, be a clearly articulated expectation, a shared purpose, a goal, and a standard.

us. Physicians, nurses, and other professional clinicians have a clinical and ethical responsibility to learn the relational proficiencies necessary to connect with their patients.

We can teach skills for connecting and we can share knowledge about what it takes, but for the actual connection to occur it requires each of us as individuals to develop our ability to be fully present, to recognize and let down our defenses, and to be willing to really see the other human being.

Accumulated Wisdom on the Therapeutic Relationship

There is an abundance of literature, research, theory, and time-tested wisdom on the topic of what comprises therapeutic and compassionate care. While this book ultimately aims to add to that existing wisdom, it could not do so without our first having taken in that wisdom, reflected on it, and tested it in our own practices.

In this section we offer the views of clinicians and authors—including philosophers, psychologists, physicians, and nurses—who have influenced our thinking and work. Some of them have contributed to the theory behind compassionate care, and others have helped to paint a picture of what the therapeutic relationship looks like in practice and/or the implications for care when it is absent.

Sidney Jourard

Sidney Jourard, a noted psychologist and author of the classic psychology text *The Transparent Self* (1971), writes that people in Western societies have chosen a path of concealment, hiding behind our roles and

A person can attain health only insofar as the person is able to be himself.

functions, rather than a path of openness and authentic disclosure of ourselves as people. He proposes that concealment leads to disconnection and isolation, a route that can result in sickness, conflict, misunderstanding, and alienation.

In *The Transparent Self*, Jourard explores the implications of what in 1971 was considered a novel premise: that a person can attain health only insofar as the person is able to be himself.

While *The Transparent Self* addresses a human way of being for people in all walks of life, Jourard also specifically addresses the importance of authentic therapeutic relationships between patients and "helpers and healers" (p. 179). He proposes that stereotyped interpersonal behavior patterns—that is, the taught or prescribed bedside manner—are intended to control the patient and to limit the professional's exposure to "threatening patterns of behavior" from the patient (p. 181). In a paradigm that leaves authenticity behind, the patient's negative emotions are suppressed whenever possible. In this scenario, where neither the patient nor the caregiver is permitted to be authentic, Jourard suggests that both are at risk of the very sort of disconnection that can result in alienation and compassion fatigue.

In Jourard's observations of care in hospitals in the late 1960s and early 1970s, he noted that physicians and nurses had been taught to use the bedside manner as a shield between themselves and their patients. The bedside manner while making rounds, he observed, was characterized by clinicians rushing in and out of the rooms, with charts in hand, standing (sometimes near the door) rather than sitting, performing rituals such as checking equipment, studying charts, and asking closed-ended and carefully targeted questions that were designed to elicit one or two-word answers. Jourard noted that physicians' bedside manners often conveyed a sense of "self-assurance and omniscience" and that the underlying rationale was "to give patients confidence" (p. 179).

Jourard describes nurses as possessing a "peculiar kind of inauthentic behavior that does more harm than good" (p. 179). He writes:

> The bedside manner appears to be something which the nurse puts on when she dons her uniform.
>
> I was in a room interviewing a patient informally about his background and current preoccupations, and on several occasions nurses entered the room to perform nursing functions. This man was seriously ill and had much on his mind, but his nurses came in talking cheerfully and did not cease the cheerful discourse until they had left. . . .
>
> I later asked the nurses to tell me about Mr. Jones. One nurse replied, "Oh he's a nice fellow." The other told me, "He's O.K., though sometimes he's a bit difficult." I asked both of them if they had any idea of what Mr. Jones had on his mind, and each said that so far as she knew, he was cheerful most of the time. (pp. 179-180)

It's notable that his observations in hospital settings were made more than forty years ago, because they contradict the perception voiced by many health care professionals today that caring and connection used to be the norm and that it's only in the last few decades or so that technology and cost constraints have interfered with connection. We are not suggesting that Jourard's observations represent the norm today. However, we believe they're worth noting so that we might pause and wonder about ways in which inauthentic interaction may be happening today. In the workshops we facilitate, health care professionals report that in order to manage time or in moments of high stress, they sometimes slip into less authentic, scripted communications and rote activities. Additionally, some customer service programs in health care organizations promote prescribed behaviors and scripting, which may have the unintended consequence of diminishing authentic and therapeutic interactions (Bush, 2011). While the goal is to improve the patient experience, we think Jourard's observations are evidence of the dark side of programmatic approaches to human relationships. He writes:

> No self-respecting physician or nurse would overlook such vital information as the patient's temperature, blood pressure, and other physical signs of progress or regress with respect to recovery. Yet, the bedside manner is nicely designed to exclude a highly important source of information that has much pertinence to the optimum response of the patient to treatment. I have reference here to information which can only be obtained through the patient's verbal disclosure of what is on his mind. Just as thermometers and sphygmomanometers reveal something about the state of the patient's body, so does verbal self-disclosure reveal something about the state of the patient as a whole person. (p. 182)

Jourard's nuanced view of the bedside manner helps us understand that prescribed interpersonal behavior interferes with the healing aims of the caregivers. It also serves clinicians as "a means of coping with the anxieties engendered by repeated encounters with suffering, demanding patients" (p. 181). He suggests that nurses have developed their own unique armor through trial and error in order to permit themselves to care for people without the disturbing feelings of "pity, anger, inadequacy, or insecurity" (p. 181). The latent function of the bedside manner is to "reduce the probability that patients will behave in ways that are likely to threaten the professional person" (p. 181).

The latent function of the bedside manner is to "reduce the probability that patients will behave in ways that are likely to threaten the professional person."

The theoretical premise that we're treating the whole person as opposed to treating solely the body has unanimous acceptance in health care. But Jourard challenges us to remember what it looks like in practice to care for that whole person. In a voice as modern as anyone writing about the health care profession today, Sidney Jourard advocates for a clinical practice grounded in honesty, authenticity, and conscious self-disclosure. Such a practice allows us to connect with our shared humanity, to feel and express compassion, and to gain greater understanding about the state of the patient as a whole being—body, mind, and spirit. Our care is thus more purposeful and effective.

Dean Ornish

Dean Ornish, a well-known cardiologist and author, believes that the lack of love, intimacy, and relationship is at the root of what makes us sick and that the presence of these elements in our lives is what makes us well.

In his book, *Love and Survival: The Scientific Basis for the Healing Power of Intimacy* (1997), Ornish reviews scientific evidence that supports his belief that love and intimacy are perhaps "the most powerful factors in health and illness—even though these ideas are largely ignored by the medical profession" (p. 20). Clearly, human connection is essential to healing; indeed, touch is essential to our survival. Ornish maintains that "lack of human contact can lead to profound isolation and illness—and even death" (p. 139).

Ornish cites evidence of this in two experiments, one ancient and one contemporary, which reveal the importance of human connection to survival and healing. He describes a horrifying experiment conducted by 13th century German emperor Frederick II to find out what would happen to children's language if they were raised without hearing anyone talk to them. To test this, the emperor took several newborn babies from their parents and placed them under the care of nurses who were forbidden to talk to them. The babies never learned a language because they died. They could not live without connection (Ornish, 1997, p. 139). He also describes a study by the Touch Research Institute in Miami in which premature babies were given three loving massages a day for ten days; these babies gained weight 47% faster than those not receiving the additional human touch. The babies receiving such significant human connection also left the hospital six days sooner, at a cost savings of $10,000 per child (Field, 1995).

As a scientist himself, Ornish both respects the scientific process and acknowledges its limitations, noting, "What is most meaningful often cannot be measured. What is verifiable may not necessarily be what is most important" (p. 4). While we do not have the ability to measure what is most meaningful—things such as human connection, therapeutic touch, and even love—Ornish maintains that our valuing of those experiences should not be diminished. We can learn about what is meaningful only by listening to the stories of those having the experience, as they are our greatest teachers.

Ornish (1997) reminds us that the most profound healing element of all is love. He writes:

> Techniques can be useful, but they are limited. I am finding that I have a choice in every moment to keep my heart open or closed, to live in love or in fear. More than any specific practice, I have found that maintaining this awareness of choice is the most important factor in keeping an open heart, for every action, every thought, every moment contains the potential for bringing us closer to either connection and healing or isolation and suffering. The direction is not inherent in the actions themselves but rather in the intentionality and motivation behind the actions. (p. 99)

Some may question whether love has any place in a professional setting, but we contend that where there is human suffering—the need of one in distress calling to one who is in a position to listen, understand, and truly see the other in need—love is what overrides every other possible factor to remind us that we are inexorably connected. In professional settings, it's more common than not to call this quality compassion, and yet it's worth pausing and wondering how our practice—indeed, how we as individuals—would be affected if we, like Ornish, accepted that love is a fundamental attribute of human caring.

Martin Buber

The work of theologian and philosopher Martin Buber has greatly influenced the humanities and our understanding of authentic connection. Perhaps his most enduring contribution is his concept of distinguishing interpersonal relationships as either "I-It" or "I-Thou" encounters. When we have an I-Thou encounter, he says, we meet one another in authentic human connection. When we have an I-It encounter, however, we do not actually meet. Instead the "I" merely encounters the other as an "It"—as an object rather than as another being. I-Thou is a relationship of mutuality, reciprocity, and shared humanity, whereas I-It is a relationship of separateness, detachment, and objectification of the other (Buber, 1958). Balancing large numbers of patients, and doing so within the context of institutions, makes us particularly susceptible to I-It encounters. If we are not intentional in seeing the other as a person we can easily slip into a detached I-It interaction which dehumanizes the other as well as ourselves.

When we are viewing people as objects we are not inclined to be open, available, and curious about who they are and what matters to them. We may, instead, see them merely as part of our workload. The I-It relationship accomplishes two things: it protects us from experiencing our own vulnerability, and it helps us control the interaction and manage the responses of the other to achieve our preconceived aims. The I-It relationship may appear to require less from us; however, over time such detached interactions diminish the self as well as the other. The I-Thou relationship requires that we be authentic in our interaction and have the desire to truly understand the other. Because it invites us to be human, it continually nourishes our humanity.

> *Because the I-Thou relationship invites us to be human, it continually nourishes our humanity."*

C. Terry Warner

C. Terry Warner, a professor of philosophy and founder of the Arbinger Institute, expanded upon Buber's concept of what it means to meet in an authentic encounter by distinguishing two ways of being with others: what he calls a *responsive* (I-You) way of being or a *resistant* (I-It) way of being (Warner, 2001). His work is grounded in the assumption that "to the immature, other people are not real" (p. 49).

Whether we choose the responsive or resistant way of being with others depends on our level of emotional maturity in that moment. When we interact from a more mature, secure, open way of being, we see the other as a person—having needs, values, and experiences which are all as legitimate as our own. We are compassionate, curious, and naturally responsive. We meet the other person from an I-You perspective. However, when we relate from a less mature, defensive, judgmental, or closed way of being, we see the other as an object—as not real—and therefore as something to be worked on, to be managed, to be worked around, or perhaps even as invisible and irrelevant. We do not meet the other person, but rather interact from an I-It perspective and have a resistant way of being (Arbinger, 2006).

The implications of understanding the two ways of being are significant for our care of people. Being conscious of the two ways of being—and recognizing that we tend to move continually from one way of being to the other and back again, usually quite unconsciously—helps us to notice when we are objectifying another through our language, our busyness, our focus on tasks rather than persons, or when we are caught up in our own agenda in such a way that the other person becomes irrelevant. By being conscious, by simply noticing, we may be able to mindfully shift our way of being and experience a responsive, authentic I-You encounter (Warner, 2001).

Carl Rogers

Carl Rogers is the founder of the humanistic approach to psychology. He is known for person-centered therapy in which the self is viewed as a therapeutic tool. He views individuals as existing in a continually changing world of experience of which they are the center. Individuals react to their experience based on their unique perceptions and realities. When individuals experience illness or trauma, their responses and capacity to cope are uniquely defined by who they are. Person-centered care would thus begin by seeking to understand the meaning of the experience through the eyes of the individual (Rogers, 1951).

Rogers, like Jourard and Warner, focuses on our capacity as caregivers to recognize and differentiate the personhood of the person for whom we are caring from our own personhood as we render care. This consciousness of individual personhood facilitates our ability to be present, curious, and open with

During times of crisis our world becomes constricted and focused on our own experience—our own pain, our own suffering, our fear of disability, our fear of dying.

40

others without having to hide behind the armor of inauthentic communication and actions.

Rogers' tenet that we all see ourselves as the center of the world is worth noting. During times of crisis our world becomes constricted and focused on our own experience—our own pain, our own suffering, our fear of disability, our fear of dying. Other aspects of our lives fade away, and what is happening to us now becomes our world. Remembering this can help us as caregivers to remember the importance of focusing on the person (and loved ones) needing care. Their agenda, their world, trumps ours. This means, however, that we are called as clinicians to do something truly extraordinary. As human beings we have an innate tendency to see ourselves as the center of the world, but as clinicians we are asked to suspend that tendency in order to put the patient's needs first. That means that no matter how close we appear to fall on the *selfless server* end of the continuum, it takes consciousness, it takes practice, and it takes discipline to be in therapeutic relationship with another.

Jean Watson

Jean Watson's *Theory of Human Caring* (1988) guides much of the caring practice of nurses and other clinicians throughout the world. Watson is the founder of the Center for Human Caring and a leader in human caring research and theory development. She describes the transpersonal caring moment as a "human-to-human relationship which transcends each individual resulting in a deeper/higher consciousness for both" (p. 115).

She emphasizes that caring is not constrained by time, but rather that caring can happen in a moment.

Watson defines the caring moment as a "transpersonal caring relationship" in which the person caring and the person receiving care feel a connection with each other. Through this connection new possibilities for healing are opened (p. 118).

Kristen Swanson

Kristen Swanson builds on Watson's framework and brings caring theory into practice. Her theory is based on research with patients, families, and caregivers who have defined what is most essential in the caring relationship. In her 1991 article, *Empirical Development of a Middle Range Theory of Caring*, Swanson describes five caring processes that can inform therapeutic practice for all clinical disciplines.

1. **Maintaining Belief:** Maintaining a fundamental belief in persons and their capacity to make it through events and transitions and face the future with meaning. Dimensions include having faith, maintaining a hope-filled attitude, and going the extra mile for the patient.

2. **Knowing:** Striving to understand an event as it has meaning in the life of the other—understanding the lived realities of those served. Dimensions include avoiding assumptions, centering on the other, thoroughly assessing, and seeking cues and expertise from the other.

3. **Being with:** Being emotionally present to the other. Dimensions include being there, enduring, listening, attending, disclosing, and not burdening.

4. **Doing for:** Doing for the other what they would do for themselves if it were possible. Dimensions include preserving dignity, protecting, comforting, and performing competently.

5. **Enabling/Informing:** Facilitating the other's passage through life transitions and unfamiliar events. Dimensions include explaining, informing, generating options, supporting, advocating, validating, and anticipating and preparing for future needs.

Swanson offers us an attainable, practical framework that intersects philosophy, psychology, theory, and practice.

Rachel Naomi Remen

Rachel Naomi Remen is a clinical professor at the University of California San Francisco School of Medicine and a cofounder and medical director of the Commonweal Cancer Help Program. She is recognized as one of the earliest pioneers in bringing human caring and healing to medical practice. She is also one of the first physicians to develop a psychological approach to helping people cope with life-threatening illnesses. This approach includes helping patients take the lead in educating their physicians about their response to their illness and their emotional needs (Remen, 1989).

Like Ornish, Remen (1989) believes that we learn best by listening to one another's stories. She credits her own experience living with Crohn's disease for informing this perspective. She states that the gift of her illness has been to help her understand the illness experiences of patients and what it means to support their healing and their dying. Remen (2002), like Jourard, Warner, Ornish, Rogers, Watson, and Swanson, emphasizes the importance of being real, authentic, and even loving, in our relationships with those in our care:

> *Many of us don't know that our love matters. We are a technological culture, so we think that we are supposed to be able to fix people's problems. Or we think there is a "right" thing to say. People want to be comforting, but they don't know how to do that. What I have discovered is that the simple human*

connection is what matters. Nobody expects you to fix their lymphoma or breast cancer, but people expect or hope that their suffering really matters to you. All that's needed is to say, "I heard about your illness, I am so sorry." Just say it and really mean it; say it from your heart. There is nothing more powerful. I remember one of the most profound things that ever happened to me when I was young, in the midst of my really severe suffering with my illness, was when this person came to me and said, "You know, I heard that it's been hard for you. I'm so sorry." Then their eyes filled with tears. I knew my life mattered. I knew that they cared about me. I felt strengthened to go on. They didn't fix a thing about me; they were just real. Some of us feel being real isn't enough. We think we are supposed to be an expert and have the right words and the right answer. We are the right answer! (p. 1)

Remen's work is a call for loving connection. She is talking about presence and authenticity and the idea that there is simply no substitute for them if healing is our goal. She also points out that lovingly witnessing and affirming another's pain and suffering can have a profound impact on a person's ability to find strength and to cope, validating Watson's theory that caring can happen in a moment.

Summary of Scholars on Human Caring

Sidney Jourard (psychologist)	Promotes a "human way of being" and emphasizes the importance of caregivers having honest, authentic, and self-disclosing interactions with patients and their loved ones. Challenges prescribed interpersonal behavior because it interferes with the healing aims of the caregivers. (Jourard, 1971)

Martin Buber (philosopher)	Distinguishes human relationships as I-Thou or I-It. The I-Thou relationship is one of mutuality, reciprocity, and shared humanity, whereas I-It is a relationship of separateness, detachment, and objectification of the other. (Buber, 1958)
C. Terry Warner (philosopher)	Builds on Buber's philosophy and identifies responsive and resistant ways of being with others. In the responsive way of being we connect with compassion and curiosity. In the resistant way of being we do not connect because we see others as obstacles, vehicles to achieve our means, or as being irrelevant. (Warner, 2001; Arbinger, 2006)
Dean Ornish (cardiologist)	Describes the importance of touch, connection, and love to our very survival. Provides a scientific imperative to touch, connect, and care with compassion. Laments our inability to "measure what is most meaningful"—things such as human connection, therapeutic touch, and even love—while asserting their inherent value to the experience of healing. Asserts also that we must learn about what is meaningful by listening to the stories of those having the experience, as they are our greatest teachers. (Ornish, 1997)
Carl Rogers (psychologist)	Known for person-centered therapy and the view of the self as a therapeutic tool. When individuals experience illness or trauma, their responses and capacity to cope are uniquely defined by who they are and the experiences they've had. Person-centered care begins by seeking to understand the meaning of the experience through the eyes of the individual. (Rogers, 1951)

Jean Watson (nurse)	Developed the theory of human caring. "Caring is not constrained by time, but can happen in a moment." Watson defines the caring moment as a "transpersonal caring relationship" in which the person caring and the person receiving care feel a connection with each other. Through this connection, new possibilities for healing are opened. (Watson, 1988)
Kristen Swanson (nurse)	Developed a practice-based theory of caring that applies to clinicians in all disciplines. Processes and actions necessary for being in a caring relationship include: maintaining belief in the capacity of the person to find meaning in their experience; seeking to understand the meaning of the illness through the eyes of the person experiencing it; being present and emotionally accessible; doing for the person those things that they would do for themselves if able; and facilitating their passage through the illness experience by guiding, informing, and advocating. (Swanson, 1993)
Rachel Naomi Remen (oncologist)	Emphasizes the importance of being authentic, honest, and present when caring for a person. She boldly lifts up the importance of love in the experience of the patient, saying that love makes healing possible. Remen encourages her fellow caregivers to believe that they have what it takes to be in a therapeutic relationship. (Remen, 1989, 2002)

The congruence among the contributions of these key scholars and others leads us to summarize with these fundamental truths about human caring and the therapeutic relationship.

A therapeutic relationship exists when:

- People know that they are seen as unique persons, as evidenced by sustained eye contact, authentic communication, and the clinician remembering what is most important to them.

- People are given the opportunity to be partners in their care; they are given information and explanations that fully prepare them to make appropriate decisions about their treatment and care.

- People perceive that they are being touched with care and kindness.

- People can see by the actions taken that they are being listened to and heard.

- People perceive that the magnitude of their illness or injury is recognized and respected.

- People are encouraged to feel a sense of hope and possibility by those who recognize and respect the magnitude of their illness or injury.

- People perceive that they are being treated with dignity and that caregivers will seek to preserve their dignity when conferring about them as well as with them.

- People are supported to cope with and find meaning in their illness.

- People feel safe and know that they will not be abandoned.

A New Mindset that Supports the Therapeutic Relationship

While the scholarship we've summarized for you in the previous pages—as well as the scholarship of countless other contributors to the creation and refinement of the therapeutic relationship—has been and will continue to be invaluable to us in our practice, we'd like to offer an additional framework for thinking, being, and doing within the therapeutic relationship. We'd like to introduce a mindset that we believe to be extremely effective in helping clinicians remain intentionally therapeutic with the people in their care.

Here's why a mindset is so important: we each have a set of long-practiced thoughts that influence who we are, what we do, and what we believe is being done to us. These long-practiced thoughts become our default thoughts as our brains create deep neural pathways that make these thoughts easier and easier to think. That means that the thoughts we've practiced the longest and most frequently are the thoughts that comprise our current mindset. Depending upon what your current mindset is, this could be good news or bad news. But no matter what thought patterns are now most active in your experience, you're not stuck with them. We can create and habitualize new thoughts, and if we integrate them and use these new thoughts long enough, they will become our new mindset.

One of the primary purposes of this book is to introduce a way of thinking that will foster the highest possible level of authentic human-to-human connection between clinicians and the people in their care. If we mindfully go to thoughts of connection when we're feeling disconnected (tired, stressed, thwarted, frustrated, overwhelmed), over time, these new thoughts of connection will determine how we view our experience. Our intention is to provide a way of thinking that supports your ability to see your patients as human beings who desire and deserve human connection—people who, in their vulnerable state, hunger to be seen as people perhaps as much as they hunger for a cure.

The way of thinking that we're offering in support of the therapeutic relationship comprises these simple practices which will be summarized briefly here, illustrated in Figure 1.2, and amplified in depth over the next four chapters:

Presence through Attunement	Presence is created through understanding the science of attunement. Presence becomes the container in which the therapeutic relationship occurs.
Wondering, Following, Holding	These three practices are ways of thinking, ways of being, and ways of acting. They facilitate an authentic, healing connection.

FIGURE 1.2: Therapeutic Practice

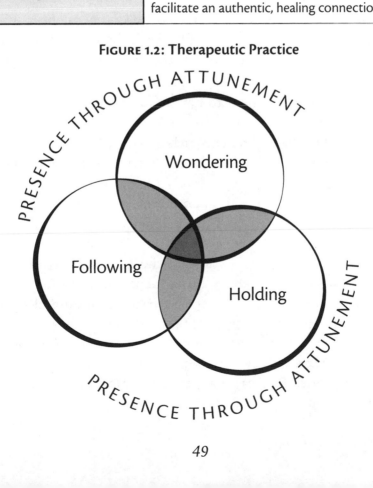

Presence through Attunement

To be present means to be consciously attuned to the person before you. Remen (1996) describes this kind of attuned presence as being "seen by the heart" (p. 149). It happens when you see the other, listen to and hear the other, and, for the moment, give your undivided attention to the one or ones in your care. It's a state that you have no doubt experienced, although it's also likely that it's a state that leaves you when the concerns of your mind and other demands of the moment become dominant. It is difficult to remain present, especially under pressure and time constraints. In the next chapter we will offer some science, some knowledge, some case studies, and some practical tips that will help you achieve greater presence through conscious attunement.

Attunement is a feeling of harmony or oneness with another being; it is both a way of being and a way of doing. It's the experience of focusing on another person with openness and acceptance.

In order for attunement to happen between a clinician and a patient, the clinician must be emotionally available to, and authentically interested in, the patient. In a clinical setting the word attunement suggests a level of connection, even if temporary, that leads the patient to resonate with the clinician and the clinician to resonate with the patient. Attunement takes focus and persistence, and it is nurtured when a clinician

When you are attuned to your patient, the patient experiences that you are truly present, and he or she feels emotionally safe.

intentionally co-constructs an experience with the patient and family. When you are attuned to your patient, the patient experiences that you are truly present, and he or she feels emotionally safe. This can happen over time, and it can also happen very quickly.

Attunement is also the immeasurable yet completely perceivable container that encompasses the three practices: wondering, following, and holding.

Wondering, Following, and Holding

The practices of wondering, following, and holding bring the therapeutic relationship to life. Each of them describes a way of interacting with patients (doing), but they are also a mindset and a way of being.

High quality care is achieved through a full connection and partnership with the patient and the patient's family. It is the patient and family who will ultimately teach us what they need and what will help them move most effectively toward their healing and recovery. Wondering, following, and holding are the practices that help us tune in to the vital information that only our patients can give us. These practices help us to keep our care on the mark as they offer us three distinct ways to become and remain present, accessible, and connected to our patients.

Wondering is a state of mind characterized by curiosity, openness, and acceptance—a joyful not-knowing and an intentional elimination of our own agenda. Wondering is supported by:

- becoming empty;

- using wide eyes;

- listening and watching with curiosity;

- noticing and suspending judgment; and

- purposefully eliminating all barriers to the above.

Following is a series of intentional acts that demonstrate devotion on the part of the clinician to being led and taught by the patient and family. Following is supported by:

- allowing each utterance of the caregiver to flow out of—and show respect for and acknowledgement of—the last thing the patient or family member said;

- allowing each act of caregiving to be consistent with what the patient or family member has taught us;

- consciously deciding to be guided by the patient's perspective, which requires knowledge of the patient's history, culture, and stories; and

- giving careful attention to the body language, touch, voice tone, and words of both the patient and the self, noticing the continuous feedback loop, and revising caregiver behaviors as required.

Holding is a conscious decision to lift up, affirm, and dignify that which the patient or family member has taught, resulting in intense focus on the patient or family member while treasuring both the information and the person. Holding creates a safe haven for patients. Holding is supported by:

- keeping confidences as needed and appropriate;

- remembering, in specific acts of care, that which has been learned about the patient, family, culture, and history;

- speaking of and writing about the patient and family—at change of shift report, in the hall, in notes—with dignity and an eagerness to transmit treasured information;

- keeping the patient informed about what is going on now and what is coming next; and

- being a steady and nonjudgmental presence even in the face of strong emotional responses.

As clinicians wonder with and about their patients, new and important information comes forward that would have been missed in a culture in which assumptions, tasks and/or agendas drive the care.

As clinicians follow their patients, individualized care plans are devised that take into consideration exactly what the patient is willing and able to do and what the family is willing and able to support, resulting in greater adherence to the plan for recovery and aftercare.

As clinicians hold their patients, both patients and their families feel seen and safe, which enhances their overall experience of care and puts them in the right conditions for healing.

Summary of Key Thoughts

- If you treat patients with kindness and dignity, they see it and they respond to it.

- Your dignity, your mission, and your values are what you bring to the bedside. Only with your consent can anyone take them away from you.

- The purpose of the therapeutic relationship is to promote, guide, and support the healing of another person through knowledgeable and authentic connection.

- Just as it would never be thought acceptable that a clinician would fail to be technically proficient, it can never be thought acceptable that a clinician be permitted to lack relational proficiency.

- The act of therapeutic connection is not owned by any one profession. The responsibility to offer care to another human being is something we all share no matter what discipline we practice. This striving to create connection in the service of care gives us a common purpose that unites us as health care professionals.

- The therapeutic relationship exists within a structure in which the technical aspects of care are intentionally balanced with the relational aspects of care. When this vital balance is maintained, patients feel cared for and clinicians thrive in their work.

- In the therapeutic relationship the needs of the person receiving care are of overriding concern, and the needs of the clinician are intentionally attended to elsewhere.

- The therapeutic relationship facilitates three key capacities of the person(s) being cared for:

  - to cope with their circumstances,

  - to understand the meaning of the illness or injury in their lives, and

  - to take ownership for their own healing and follow-through.

- The taught or prescribed (stereotypical) bedside manner tends to control the patient interaction and limits the clinicians' ability to learn what is important to the patient and what is important for healing the whole person.

- Human contact and love are both essential to survival.

- I-Thou is a relationship of mutuality, reciprocity, connection, and shared humanity, whereas I-It is a relationship of separateness, detachment, disconnection, and objectification of the other.

Similarly, one's way of being with others can be described as either responsive or resistant.

- As human beings we see ourselves as the center of the world, but as caregivers we are asked to suspend that tendency in order to put the patient's needs first.

- Caring is not constrained by time; caring can happen in a moment.

- Attunement is a feeling of harmony or oneness with another; it is both a way of being and way of doing. It's the experience of focusing on another person with openness and acceptance.

- When you are attuned to your patient, the patient experiences that you are truly present and he feels emotionally safe.

- As clinicians wonder with and about their patients, new and important information comes forward that would have been missed in a culture in which assumptions, tasks, and/or agendas drive the care.

- As clinicians follow their patients, individualized care plans are devised that take into consideration exactly what the patient is willing and able to do and what the family is willing and able to support, resulting in greater adherence to the plan for recovery and aftercare.

- As clinicians hold their patients, both patients and their families feel seen and safe, which enhances their overall experience of care and puts them in the right conditions for healing.

Reflection

- What struck you about Maria's story, "The Cloak"? In what ways have you experienced similar dynamics with patients in your care? Were you able to stay focused on care? If so, what helped you? If not, what disrupted your care? What did you learn from the experience?

- Which of the scholars/authors on human caring most inspires your understanding of the therapeutic relationship? Why? Who most challenges your thinking? Why?

- What do you think about Sidney Jourard's description of authentic vs. prescribed or scripted interaction? What surprises you about his observations? What challenges you? To what extent do you think his observations hold true today and in what ways? Name one or two actions that you will take in your practice to strengthen the authentic therapeutic connection you have with patients and their families.

- In what way do you think our various roles and/or clinical disciplines affect the purpose and depth of the therapeutic relationship?

- Reflect on this statement: "The act of therapeutic connection is not owned by any one profession. The responsibility to offer care to another human being is something we all share. This striving to create connection in the service of care gives us a common purpose that unites us as health care professionals." Do you agree with this thought? If yes, why? If no, why not? If this were a dominant belief in your health care culture, what would be the effect on interdisciplinary relationships, collaboration, and care for patients?

- Psychologist Carl Rogers suggested that we are "called as clinicians to do something truly extraordinary. As human beings we have an innate tendency to see ourselves as the center of the world, but we are asked to suspend that tendency in order to put the patient's needs first." What mindset does it take to consistently put the needs of the patient and family first? What challenges you most? What helps most?

- Reflect on this statement by Jean Watson: "Caring is not constrained by time; caring can happen in a moment." What does this mean to you and to your practice?

- What story about your clinical experience do you find yourself sharing most often? What is it about that story that makes it worth sharing? How do you feel when you share it?

- Reflect on what you were taught about being in relationship with patients and their family members. Notice how what you learned is visible or not in your current practice. What are you most proud of about your practice? What do you want to strengthen or change?

- If there was one thing you'd like to remember in every therapeutic encounter, what would it be? Why?

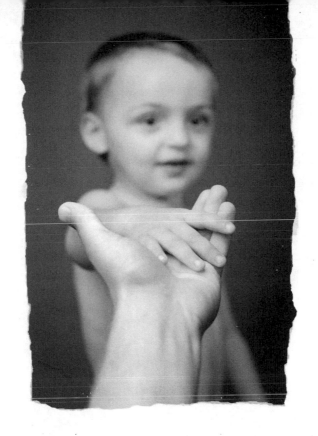

Chapter Two

Presence through Attunement

Let others see their own greatness
when looking in your eyes.

—MOLLIE MARTI, PSYCHOLOGIST AND PROFESSOR

*I*t's where everything begins.

It's a moment few of us can remember, but none of us can forget: the first time another living being looks into our eyes. We are seen. We encounter another.

We are seconds out of the uterus where there has been a kind of kinetic attunement, as mother and baby attend to each other's movements; a biological attunement that is embedded in our cellular memories, as mother and baby respond to each other's hormonal signals; and an emotional attunement, as mother and baby cue into each other's changing moods.

Now, out here in the too-bright lights of this outside world, our eyes meet, and through those eyes, souls speak to each other. The mother's or father's eyes communicate, "I see you. I know who you are. I claim you. You are now outside, but I will not forsake you. I will keep you safe."

The baby's eyes, at least in the imagination of the astonished parents, seem to communicate, "Yes, I know you, too. We have been together for some time now. I will search every square millimeter of your face again and again in the coming months, and I will come to know it as my source for danger signals, my reassurance of safety, my cue that I am loved."

We are present with one another, and that presence heals things in us that we didn't even know were broken.

We are present with one another, and that presence—the eye-to-eye, deeply-breathed connection in which at least one being is in calm, silent wonderment of the other—heals things in us that we didn't even know were broken. Here the stage is set for how safe and how loved and how self-confident and how capable of managing danger and worry this little baby will be for the rest of his life.

When there is mis-attunement, though, another kind of life begins. When the mother is unconscious or the father is absent or either parent is drunk or depressed or deeply disappointed, presence is missing, and those feelings are also communicated to the baby. The baby responds with efforts to awaken his parents' love or to regulate parents' moods or to enliven frozen expressions. For a while the baby tries hard, and then he begins to give up a bit. He will try again later.

The Science of Attunement: We Learned it When We Were Small

Attunement with another human being is one of our earliest quests. It seems likely that evolution is at the heart of it: we connect with each other in the beginning as part of a biological imperative to survive. Where there is deep connection between a baby and a primary caregiver, food is more likely to arrive, protection is more likely to be forthcoming, unkindness and violence are less likely to enter the picture, and survival is more likely to be assured (Blum, 2002; Bowlby, 1969).

A scientific phenomenon in infant development, poorly understood until recently, is the way in which the caregiver's attunement with the baby contributes to the infant's capacity to regulate his own inner states. Actually, our grandmothers probably understood this very well. They knew that an upset daddy would usually have trouble calming an upset baby. They knew that babies respond to particular vocal sounds, timbres, and rhythms, as well as to the nuances of parental facial expressions, the specific quality of parental movements, and even to unseen but clearly experienced phenomena such as parental mood.

Science has now caught up and has documented the experience of co-regulation that occurs when any two individuals are well attuned. Babies notice and internally experience the mental state of their primary caregiver and begin to attune to it. In the process, the baby's neurology begins to connect to that of the primary caregiver, giving the caregiver a strange capacity to actually regulate—without ever lifting a finger, so to speak—the mood and movements and affect of the baby. Slowly the baby, carefully attuned to the parent, begins to pick up on this capacity and develops the ability to regulate himself (Schore, 2001; Schore, 2002; Siegel, 1999). These early co-regulatory experiences set the stage for the baby's ability to soothe himself on the first day of kindergarten, to regulate his anxiety before that big speech in fifth grade, or to do self-talk when he is in agony over the loss of his first love as an adolescent.

Infants are predisposed from birth to interpret the subjective meaning of facial expressions, and they become highly motivated to communicate with their caregivers in this way. Early researchers wondered what would happen if that hunger for attuned connection was frustrated. In what were called the still-face procedures, mothers faced their infants in a laboratory, and initially interacted "normally" (Gianino & Tronick, 1988; Tronick & Cohn, 1989). They were then instructed to suddenly turn "still" and unresponsive while continuing to face their babies. The infants began the most remarkable sequence of attunement-seeking behaviors—including reaching (sometimes with feet), exaggerated facial expressions, and other efforts to "reach" the affectively-flat and unresponsive mother—before taking a break, trying again, becoming agitated and dysregulated, and eventually collapsing into withdrawal and sorrow.

As we develop into adults, we learn to cope with a lack of affect or a mis-attuned affect in others, but we never get comfortable with it. It doesn't feel good to encounter it, and it doesn't feel good to offer it to others.

But what in the world does this have to do with the provision of health care in the 21st century? What does this have to do with making connections with grownups? What does this have to do with the therapeutic relationship?

We have discovered that it has everything to do with it.

The Effect of Attunement on the Patient's Experience

Away from familiar and reassuring elements of his own environment, an individual who is dropped into a foreign setting such as a hospital may feel, or actually be, dependent on his caregivers. The experience of the patient, who is often momentarily regressed and fearful, may be remarkably like the experience of the infant: searching, wondering about safety, needful of touch, needful of reassurance, needful of information about the environment, needful of one who is present and seeks to understand. While this is certainly not a call to treat adult and child patients like babies, there is something for clinicians to learn from the infant's experience of dependency and connection. There is also something to learn about the huge range of methods—many of them nonverbal—by which parents deliver reassurance, containment, and respect to their children, and by which clinicians can deliver reassurance, containment, and respect to patients and their families.

The experience of the patient when she was little, dependent, and worried may predict the sort of patient she becomes if she ever enters the health care system.

- Does she experience shame at being weak and needful because that is how she felt when she was little, resulting in a passive (or passive-aggressive) role as a recipient of health care?

- Does she experience terror at being dependent and unsure of the circumstances around her as a result of being left alone when she was little, resulting in incessant pushing of the call-button, but finds nothing done for her to be adequate?

- Did she have a mother whose attunement was so exquisite and gentle that now, as a patient, she welcomes each thing done for her as a gift and shows her gratitude because you merely said "Good morning"?

- Was her experience of mis-attunement so unsettling when she was little that she has now become defiant about ever needing anything or anybody?

Unfortunately, in fast-paced acute care settings we're not always able to gain insights into how our patients' past experiences of attunement may be affecting their ability to receive care. Still, there are some things we can do that help all of our patients to experience us as fully present and attuned to them. Patients who feel vulnerable and dependent are comforted and enjoy a greater sense of safety when clinicians are present in these ways:

- Engaging in respectful, unhurried communication while orienting our body in the same plane as the patient's body, orienting our face in the same plane as the patient's face, and making eye contact.

- Listening and giving evidence that we are listening.

- Setting aside other activities and movements for a few seconds in order to engage and listen without interruption.

- Sharing timely information about what is currently happening and what is about to happen in the patient's experience, especially during transitions.

- Giving reassurance based on the factual realities of the patient's specific condition.

- Remembering and acting on what the patient has told us is important.

- Conveying non-judging acceptance of the emotional responses of the patient and loved ones.

- Showing genuine interest in the patient and family as people.

The Effect of Attunement on the Clinician's Experience

The capacity for attunement that each of us has as a health care provider is also intimately linked with the sort of connections we made in our earliest years. Did we feel seen? Did we revel in the warm embrace—an embrace often created merely with the eyes—of another? Do we know what it feels like to experience danger or worry and then to have those feelings diminish merely as a result of physical proximity and emotional connection with a particular person? Have we, as a result, found ourselves attentive to the worries of others? Have people come to rely on our empathy with them? Who have we become as caregivers because of our own experience of attunement (or the lack thereof) as we developed into the human beings we now are? Is our presence something we find ourselves offering to our patients, or do we find that we cannot offer it?

When we are attuned to one another, these are some of the things we're more likely to do:

- Attunement causes us to notice body movement, facial expression, changes in muscle tone or respiration, and other expressions of another person's state of being.

- Attunement makes us curious about people so that we look with deep interest at others, wondering.

- Attunement draws us into rhythmic interaction—a kind of reciprocal exchange—with another person.

- Attunement allows us to more fully perceive the impact that our own presence in the room, the procedures we carry out, and our own movements and facial expressions have on the other.

- Attunement causes us to align ourselves with others, which may be evident in everything from our respiration to the next question we ask.

- Attunement means we see a person as a person rather than as an obstacle or an object or a labeled category.

- Attunement means we have a stake in the welfare of the person to whom we are attuned.

Compassion and Empathy Deepen Attunement

The word *compassion* comes from the Latin and literally means, "to suffer with." Compassion is a quality that allows us to attune to the suffering of other people and to care deeply about their suffering.

Empathy is a component of compassion which entails both the recognition of the other person's experience and a willingness to remain fully present in the face of it. It comes from a Greek root word meaning "in feeling" or "feeling into." True empathy means that we are highly attuned to what it's like to be in the person's situation, even if we ourselves have no direct experience of that situation. Empathy requires consciousness as well as an openness to receiving the person's experience without judgment.

While compassion and empathy are not quite the same thing, we think that they are nearly inseparable, and further, that they are inexorably linked to the practice of attunement. It's important to note at the outset, however, that compassion and empathy in therapeutic care are distinct from pitying or over-identifying with a person's suffering. Stephen Levine, poet, healer, and author of the book *A Year to Live* (1998), distinguishes pity from compassion in the following way: "Pity arises from meeting pain with fear. Compassion comes when you meet it with love" (p. 18).

Pity arises from meeting pain with fear. Compassion comes when you meet it with love.

— Stephen Levine

Highly attuned, compassionate care is care in which we are clearly self-differentiated as clinicians and therefore are able to lovingly keep front-of-mind our understanding of what it means to be vulnerable and ill. We feel attuned to the visceral pain of the person without becoming overwhelmed by our own emotional experience of the person's suffering. Our development as clinicians requires us to be attuned to our own emotions so that we can regulate ourselves, manage our stress, and maintain an emotional resilience that facilitates our ability to care for people in pain without losing our sense of self in the process.

It is not the slightest overstatement to say that the very survival of our species is dependent on compassionate care marked by a high level of personal attunement. As we discussed in Chapter 1, studies on the deprivation of human touch demonstrate that infants fail to thrive physically, mentally, and emotionally if they do not receive human connection and nurturing (Ornish, 1997; Field, 1995).

The same has been demonstrated with the frail and elderly, who will begin to deteriorate far more rapidly if left alone and untouched (Bush, 2001). Human compassion and empathy are as much at the heart of medicine, nursing, and the allied health professions as they are at the heart of all ethical and spiritual traditions. This is a fundamental truth, yet we sometimes struggle to keep it central to our systems and practice.

Both compassion and empathy reflect the courage it takes to enter into and stay present with another person's painful experience without retreating or trying to change or fix it. In our work, there is curing (which is sometimes possible), and there is healing (which is almost always possible to some degree). We cure diseases, not people. Healing is, conversely, something that can only take place between attuned clinicians and the people they connect with. When attuned clinicians show both compassion and empathy, a human connection of mutual vulnerability and intimacy creates a bond that may last no more than a moment but that may heal wounds that have been carried for a lifetime.

The Magic of Attunement

We suddenly feel comfortable with a complete stranger we happened to sit next to on the train. It's as if we have known each other before. We "click." We are surprised and then we become excited about how the conversation grows, the turns it takes, the humor or intimacy that characterizes it. We say things we wouldn't say to anyone except a family member, and maybe not even to them!

Later we think about the interaction. We want to tell someone: "I just ran into the nicest lady." The memory fades eventually, but the feeling of being connected, albeit very briefly, may remain.

We have connected.

An observer might say we looked like old friends, but the truth is that this connection was very much between our two brains, and it happened because each person experienced the other as present. This level of exquisite attunement which, in this case, may have happened quite naturally as a result of recognition of similarity or a moment early in the interaction in which one person felt seen or understood by the other, built on itself. The excitement of feeling attuned to another human being encouraged us to move in just a little closer, maybe even to trust a little, to want more.

Mainstream medical research now documents what we have long sensed in these situations in which we truly connect and attune to another. When there is attunement, each person begins to shape the electrical activity of the other person's brain (Siegel, 1999). They begin to co-construct a shared experience. UCLA developmental neuropsychiatrist Daniel Siegel (1999) suggests that we actually begin to enter each other's worlds, to enter each other's brains, to affect each other: " . . . [our] nonverbal signals, including facial expression, tone of voice, gestures, and timing of response, have a direct impact [on the other]" (p. 277). It is in this manner that the emotional state of the receiver is directly shaped by that of the sender. We become collaborators. We are on the same side.

This is both good news and bad news, of course. It means that deliberate attuning begets attunement, but it also means that a chaotic mind in one of us contributes to feelings of chaos in another. Consider this metaphor: You are a chemical compound, and each room you enter is a beaker containing other chemical compounds. Each time you enter a room you change its chemistry. Now ask yourself this question: When I enter a room, how do I change the chemistry in that room?

The energy in the room does change when you enter it. Sometimes it changes in an obvious way and sometimes the change is very subtle, but your entrance into a room is never without effect. You may have had the experience of a patient becoming agitated or tense and withdrawn when you entered a room; you also may have had the experience of a patient breathing easier, perhaps experiencing an actual sigh of relief upon seeing you. The patient puts forward a vibrational request to connect and asks you to answer that request. With your presence, with your eyes, with your questions (which are based on things that are meaningful to the patient) and perhaps with your touch, you find a way to connect. Presence, attunement, and co-regulation are achieved, if only for a moment or two.

More often than not, however, it's not the patient who initiates this co-construction of experience. Often it's your intentional use of self that shifts the chemistry between the two of you so that a deliberate, peaceful attunement is possible.

It's likely that you know this experience well. You take a moment outside the doorway before meeting a patient. You remember how important it is to the patient's sense of well-being that each encounter has a definite beginning, middle, and end. You set your intention to wonder on behalf of the patient, to be curious, to become open, releasing judgments and perhaps stress from the previous encounter. You are in a mode of discovery. You've changed your chemistry in those brief moments, which changes the chemistry of the patient once your chemistries begin to mix. What you're now bringing into your encounter with the patient may be vastly different from the chemical compound the two of you would have comprised just moments earlier.

As you step into the room, you bring a dose of presence with you. You bring a willingness to attune and even the conscious intention to do so. Your curiosity guides your questions, and the patient's answers and nonverbal cues determine what questions you'll ask next. Because your questions are clearly based on what the patient is giving you, you're getting truthful answers. Because you ask for clarification when you are confused, the patient feels permitted to do the same. His easy, automatic, "Yes, I'll do that," is eventually replaced by the probably much more helpful, "I'm not sure what you mean." The clinician learns about the patient. The patient feels seen and heard, and therefore, held.

You may know someone whose physical presence seems, without fail, to have a calming effect on just about everyone; all she has to do is walk into a room. The people she encounters are visibly shifted as a sort of co-regulation is achieved. Someone calm and strong walks in and, whether that person is officially in charge or not, everyone in the room breathes more deeply, shoulders relax, possibilities and solutions are seen more easily. You may even be that person.

You may or may not have a sense of exactly what it is that she brings to her encounters—nor may she, for that matter—because it may be completely natural to her. But there are observable characteristics to what she brings that we can learn and emulate: Her mind is clear of stories, labels, and preconceived notions; she's there to discover and to accept what she discovers just as it is.

Soon her eyes convey the calm, strong confidence of a person who knows that presence alone is sometimes enough and that to offer less is an affront to the dignity of another.

She breathes deeply, and when she talks with people, the experience of co-regulation gets stronger as her unwavering presence invites the presence of others. Soon, like the grandmother holding the child, her eyes convey the calm, strong confidence of a person who knows that presence alone is sometimes enough, and that to offer less is an affront to the dignity of the other.

Sometimes it's impossible to take the pain away completely, and sometimes a person truly is inconsolable, but with co-regulation, or even just co-breathing—the experience of consciously slowing your breath in order to entrain the other to a slower, calmer rhythm—clinicians can attune with their patients in such a way that their fears are calmed and their capacity to cope is enhanced, thus making the moment more endurable. This practice is easily seen in clinicians who care for women during labor and delivery, but it can be applied to any situation in which a person is experiencing anxiety or discomfort.

A Patient's Experience of Attuned Presence: Jill Bolte Taylor

Dr. Jill Bolte Taylor is a neuroanatomist who, while conducting research at Harvard Medical School's Department of Psychiatry, experienced a massive left hemisphere stroke. In her 2006 book *My Stroke of Insight*, she wrote of one part of her experience as a patient:

> *With this shift into my right hemisphere, I became empathic to what others felt. Although I could not understand the words they spoke, I could read volumes from their facial expressions and body language. I paid very close attention to how energy dynamics affected me. I realized that some people brought me energy while others took it away. One nurse was very attentive to my needs. Was I warm enough? Did I need water? Was I in pain? Naturally, I felt safe in her care. She made eye contact and was clearly providing me with a healing space. A different nurse, who never made eye contact, shuffled her feet as though she were in pain. This woman brought me a tray with milk and jello, but neglected to realize that my hands and fingers could not open the containers. I desperately wanted to consume something, but she was oblivious to my needs. She raised her voice when she spoke to me, not realizing that I wasn't deaf. Under the circumstances, her lack of willingness to connect with me scared me. I did not feel safe in her care. (pp. 74-75)*

Dr. Bolte Taylor silently pleaded for attunement. Everything at that point in her care seemed to depend on her catching the attention of her caregivers. She needed desperately for them to see her, to discover her, to find the person inside.

Here she lay, a brilliant scientist with a PhD (though it could have been any one of us) who could not begin to communicate what was wrong. Language and logical reasoning were gone. Her only hope lay in the capability of somebody to step inside her world, attune to the meager means of communication she had available, attune to her desperate hunger for information, attune to exactly the person she was at that moment: a wounded being, scared to death, unable to understand what was said to her, and terrifyingly mute.

When Dr. Bolte Taylor was unable to communicate, but hyper-able to read the energy of those who entered her room, she sensed something that most of us don't consciously sense. She saw, and was profoundly affected by, what happens to the chemistry of a room when a person enters it.

Another Patient's Experience of Attuned Presence: Marcus Engel

Marcus Engel was a freshman at Missouri State University when he lost his eyesight—indeed, most of his face—in a horrifying auto accident. He allowed Michael to write the following piece for a meditation CD for health care providers called *See Me as Person: Meditations for Sustaining Relationship-Based Care* (Trout, 2011), which was developed as a companion piece for this book. The meditation was inspired by Engel's book, *I'm Here: Compassionate Communication in Patient Care* (2010). In this piece, as well as in Marcus's book, we go inside Marcus's experience so that we can understand what it felt like to be traumatized and dependent—and into the healing power of presence and attunement.

Just Two Words

All I have are sounds:
breaking glass,
a woman screaming,
the clamor of EMS workers,
the click of a stretcher as the wheels fall into place,
a squawking CB radio.

I can't follow them.
I can't put them in order.
I can't focus on them.
They just keep happening.

Someone shouts my name,
ordering me to lie still.

I notice the taste of blood,
the warmth of a blanket,
the pieces of concrete that seem stuck to me.

I am blind.
I wasn't, a few minutes ago.
Don't ask me how I know that I am,
and that I will be
for the rest of my life.
I just do.
And now the searing pain makes its presence known
for the first time.
Hands are everywhere,
ravaging me,
cutting off my clothes,
grabbing me,
sticking me.
I must be letting them know about the pain,
because they start to pour gallons of morphine
into what's left of my body.

It does nothing for the pain,
that I can tell,
but it does make me stupid.

I slip away into . . .
sleep?

I awaken into increasing knowledge
of a pain unlike anything I could ever have imagined.
Everything is black.
Every square inch of my body has been raped.
Paparazzi flashbulb explosions of pain.

Through which I hear the voice
for the first time.
"Marcus."
She spoke my name.
"Can you hear me?"
There it is, again.
I move my head,
trying to orient to the sound.
A searing jolt slices my head back into place.
I gasp.
As I do,
the sucking sound of inhalation comes from my throat.
My throat?
Not my mouth?

Her fingers on my arm.
And then I slip away
again.

Minutes (or hours? or days?) later
I slam back into consciousness.
The fingers are still there.
And then the voice, again:
"Marcus? Can you hear me?"

With a sweetness,
and a presence
that helps me—in the midst of this cacophony of pain—
feel soft
and oriented,
she tells me there has been an accident.
I am in a place called "Barnes."

But it's the next two words that have stayed with me,
all these years later,
and that have made the sound of this young girl
sing in my mind
through countless surgeries
and horrible discoveries about what I can no longer do.
Just two words Jennifer spoke.
But they made all the difference.
"I'm here."

Perhaps what our patients want most from us is our carefully attuned presence, and even if they don't consciously know that they want it, their bodies know it. The need began before birth (Chamberlain, 1998; Nathanielsz, 2001; Neubauer & Neubauer, 1990), and it may well be what ensures that our most fundamental safety needs are met. Especially when we are fearful, the yearning for attunement—for the knowledge that

The yearning for attunement—for the knowledge that we are truly seen and are safe in the hands of one who cares—remains with us forever.

we are truly seen and are safe in the hands of one who cares—remains with us forever.

Remembering Our Capacity for Attunement

Mirror neurons were discovered quite accidentally in a lab at the University of Parma in Italy when researchers noticed that motor neurons would fire in the brain of one macaque while that animal watched another macaque move (Blakeslee, 2006; Rizzolatti, Fogassi, & Gallese, 2001). The observing animal never actually moved a muscle, but the activity of his brain made it appear that he did. The neurology of one mimicked the neurology of another.

Interestingly, this did not surprise the lead researcher who later wrote:

> We are exquisitely social creatures. Our survival depends on understanding the actions, intentions and emotions of others . . . .Mirror neurons allow us to grasp the mind of others not through conceptual reasoning but through direct simulation. By feeling, not by thinking. (Blakeslee, 2006, p. 1)

Does this suggest that evolution selects for attunement? Do we need the capacity to detect and understand the experiences of others in order to survive? Do we use our own bodies—including many hardwired parts—to engage in this survival-based but imminently sophisticated act? Is attunement, then, natural? If it is natural, perhaps attunement will come if we just get out of the way.

We get in the way of attunement when we sabotage our natural curiosity, our natural empathy, and our natural tendency to hook into the experience of another. We do this when we make assumptions, when we move too fast, focus too little, focus on the wrong things, abuse our own bodies, forget to take care of our own souls, or forget our principles in the service of the latest technology or the latest or most immediate demands of the institution. It may help us to remember, however, that the phenomenon of mirror neurons suggests that everyone with "typical" neurology has the capacity for attunement and that most of us do it automatically. It follows, then, that our patients may be attuning to us much of the time whether we are attuning to them or not. If they are tuning in to our mis-attunement, often characterized by our task-focus or our routinized actions, behaviors, and speech, they are likely to feel abandoned and fearful even when we're right there with them.

The vast majority of us learned attunement as babies. It was a gift to us. Activated were parts of our brains already hard-wired to do the job, to connect, to "read," to feel with another. What would it take to nourish that capacity now in each and every one of us?

Learning to Attune

There is no question that attunement with others is necessary in order for authentic relationships to happen. Therefore, it is also not in question whether attunement with others is essential to compassionate, person-centered care. Unfortunately, because a vast majority of our clinical education focuses on the instrumental aspects of our work, we often leave the individual clinician to sink or swim when it comes to his relationships with patients and co-workers based on whatever level of interpersonal attunement he has acquired experientially over his lifetime.

Fortunately, evidence suggests that attunement can be learned.

An inspiring example of an individual learning to attune to others under extremely adverse circumstances is found in the story of Temple Grandin. Grandin has autism, a neurological disorder that makes it extremely difficult for her to become attuned to others. People with autism often have difficulty reading the social cues and personal signals of others. They have trouble decoding social exchanges between others (e.g., "Why is that person jumping around?" or "Why is that boy sitting on that other boy?"). They do not easily read intentions or facial expressions and may not grasp others' expectations. Those closest to a person with autism sometimes have difficulty remembering that the family member or friend with autism is not brutally insensitive, as it may seem on some days, but merely doesn't catch on to the meaning of tears or why someone would want to hug them. For this reason, despite her mother's sensitivity and emotional availability, Temple Grandin had great difficulty attuning to others, and not surprisingly, she also had difficulty attuning to herself.

When someone was unkind to her she might feel it, but she would not know what she was feeling. As a result she would react with anxiety or even panic. In such moments she might find comfort in spinning or rolling on the ground, but it was many years before she could identify specifically what it was that she needed at these times. Movements like these provided a gentle pressure around her body—the missing hug which, in her case, had always been available to her but that she was neurologically predisposed to reject. It was still more years before she would learn, more through scientific study than through the more typical channels of experiential learning, to identify what she was feeling.

After finishing high school, Grandin spent a summer on her aunt's Arizona cattle ranch, and she became interested in a device used for holding cows steady while they were being inoculated. This machine held the cow between two metal panels that provided firm, gentle pressure. It was a "hug machine" for cows, and she observed that it appeared to calm them down. She attuned to the cows and to what they were experiencing. It may have been the scientific observer in her that triggered this new feeling of connection to another, but through continued observation of the cows and their full range of behaviors, she developed a deep attunement to cows. Once she was attuned to the cows, she developed an extraordinary sense for what would make them feel calm and happy.

Some time after her discovery that the hug machine had a consistently calming effect on the cows, in a moment of panic, Grandin put herself into this metal contraption and convinced her aunt to pull the levers that would administer the warm metallic hug to her own body. Always the astute observer (strange for someone with a disorder that is usually associated with lack of sensitivity to self and others, but not at all strange for a scientist), she began to notice how the machine made her feel. For perhaps the first time in her life, she was self-attuned enough to notice that her racing brain had calmed; her neurology felt regulated; her body relaxed. For the rest of the summer, Grandin, with the help of her aunt, took advantage of the calming abilities of the hugging machine (Ferguson & Jackson, 2010).

The most important point here is, of course, that Temple Grandin was not in any way predisposed to be able to attune to herself or anyone else. She learned to attune, and if she can learn to attune, so can others. Fortunately for those of us with more typical neurologies, all it takes to learn and develop our abilities to attune is a sustained commitment to some practices that will help us develop both attunement with self and attunement with others.

Erie Chapman, in his book *Radical Loving Care: Building the Healing Hospital in America* (2007), describes authentic or healing presence—what we're calling attunement—as a skill that can be developed as long as it begins with authentic intention (p. 90). Chapman contrasts healing

Presence is a skill that can be taught.

presence with "split presence," in which the caregiver is distracted by other tasks or responsibilities, and "robotic presence," in which caregivers treat the patient encounter as a transaction, signaling to the patient that he or she is more object than human being. Chapman proposes that presence is a skill that can be taught, and he suggests that we begin by reflecting on someone in our lives who personifies a healing presence—perhaps a colleague, family member, or friend. Making ourselves aware of what they do and how it makes us feel facilitates our ability to gift others with the same kind of presence. He believes that the "gift of presence is something every caregiver can cultivate" (p. 94), and in so doing, bring the sacred into the act of giving care.

Daniel Siegel, in his book *The Mindful Brain: Reflection and Attunement in the Cultivation of Well-Being* (2007), also maintains that self-attunement (which he calls intrapersonal attunement) is a teachable skill, as is our ability to be present and attuned to others (interpersonal attunement). Siegel maintains, however, that it cannot be taught as "information-giving." Instead, self-attunement is most effectively developed through an individual's commitment to reflection. In Grandin's case, for example, she did not participate in what we might think of as a typical self-reflection practice. However, as a scientist she reflected tirelessly on all of the data she observed, and it was through this reflection that she developed the ability to attune to both herself and others.

Clearly, Siegel has found, attunement is developed through deepening our knowledge and understanding of ourselves and others through mindfulness and reflection. Siegel (2007) refers to reflection as the "fourth 'R' of education" (p. 259); without reflection, part of our brain actually goes unused. "Reflection is the education that develops the prefrontal cortex of the brain"— what Siegel refers to as the "neural hub of our humanity" (p. 261). It's in this region of our brains that we deepen our personal awareness and our capacity to attune to another person. If the prefrontal cortex of our brain goes unexercised, our levels of personal awareness and our capacity to attune to others will be underdeveloped.

Conversely, when a person engages in self-reflection she develops her potential for enhanced curiosity, openness, acceptance, and love, all of which comprise the acronym coined by Siegel: COAL (2007). Siegel maintains that "the perspective of self-understanding within this COAL frame of mind can directly create ways of knowing that can be transformative" (p. 128). As we gain greater self-understanding, we grow greater self-compassion and self-acceptance, which influences us to see and experience others with greater curiosity, openness, acceptance and love—truly a transformative view of our world.

Taking a Break: Attunement Broken, Attunement Repaired

Given how much seems to ride on attunement—with respect to our own social development as well as the nuances of our relatedness to others—it may seem strange to suggest that there appears to be value in episodic breaks in attunement followed by repair. Yet we see just such patterns emerge when we carefully watch lovers, mothers and babies, those in deep conversation with each other, and even those in instrumental exchanges (passing on information, for example). While we have tried to suggest that attunement to the patient is a necessary and sometimes overlooked element in establishing a therapeutic relationship in a health care setting, it is important to note that we don't have to be perfect at it and that it is normal to take breaks from it.

A mother and baby gaze lazily into each other's eyes, perhaps during breastfeeding. Distractions are minimal (and may be ignored even when they do occur). It's as if nothing is important except what's happening right here. It's as if no one else even exists.

Yet even in this circumstance, the baby looks away. It may be for rest. It may be that he is seeking variety. It may be for only a few seconds, but he does break the gaze.

The mother does as well. She may do it at the same time her baby does, or she may choose her own time to briefly interrupt this amazing moment of attunement. They both seem to know a secret in human interaction: at some point, continuous attunement gets exhausting and stops feeling right. An unbroken stare between two adults can feel intrusive, uncomfortable, even threatening. An unbroken gaze from parent to child can start feeling like the evil eye. Continuous emotional attunement can begin to feel like too much or it can even feel like mocking.

We are built for variety. We like change. We want people to connect with us, to demonstrate with their eyes and their movements and their attention that they are with us. But the power of such attunement diminishes over time if there is no break, no interruption, no chance to regroup.

What we seek in connections with others is not continuous attunement, but a series of episodes of attunement intermixed with breaks in attunement followed by repair (re-approach, reengagement), and then resumption of attunement (Brazelton & Cramer, 1990).

Healthy adults in relationship with each other figure out these rhythms based on their individual and separate needs. Completely silent and sometimes unconscious negotiations establish the patterns, and then adjustments are made depending on changing mood or maturing needs. They figure out how much to be together, how much of that together-time can be at what level of attunement, and how much of it can be just time in proximity with each other without much intimacy or contact. When two people get this right, they find that even moments during which they are barely looking at or talking with each other can feel quite intimate.

Less healthy dyads may find that they must destabilize the whole relationship from time to time, in an unconscious effort to regulate intimacy, to modulate attunement. One partner may pick a fight just for the chance to "look away" (or be away). Even in these extreme situations, repair often follows (usually with a major surge in apparent emotional intimacy), although sometimes at the price of destabilization and mistrust.

The take-away, for those of us who value the therapeutic relationship, is this: We don't have to be perfect at attunement. We are all built to tolerate periods in which there are breaks or lapses in it. We are even able to tolerate the feelings of aloneness, worry, and fear that sometimes accompany such breaks or lapses, as long as repair—beginning with re-engagement and then restoration of attunement—occurs before too much time has passed.

Mindful Attunement throughout the Day

The following meditation was written by Michael for the meditation CD *See Me as a Person* (Trout, 2011) and is based on Siegel's COAL framework. This meditation can be used in groups and by individuals in order to become focused on the humanity of our patients and families as the work day begins.

My Caregiving Stance for Today

Just for this one moment
let me look upon this person
with Curiosity
Openness
Acceptance
and Love.

Let me imagine his eyes before they filled with fear,
before her gaze became obscured by worry,

before they became faraway eyes,
searching for something I can't see.

Let me picture this person before the reason she came into my care
became the only thing.

Let me imagine that those eyes once saw things
of beauty, and grace, and joy, and hope.
Let me imagine that this person,
just for this moment,
needs for me to remember where he came from,
and all she has done in her life,
and all the people who have loved him,
and still do.

I can't fix it all.
Just for this one day, tho',
let me do my little part:
Curiosity
Openness
Acceptance
Love.

Thich Nhat Hanh, a Buddhist monk and prolific writer, teaches mindful living as a disciplined practice. Like Siegel, he says that through this disciplined practice we can be freed from the grip of reactivity, defensiveness, fear, and anger, enhancing our ability to be present in the moment (Nhat Hanh, 1992).

While he strongly encourages us to engage in formal sitting meditation practice, he also proposes that we can be mindful as we move through our day by incorporating some very simple practices. As these practices become integrated into our daily activities, we develop a greater capacity for being present and responding with compassion. For example, we may use the ringing of a phone as a cue to breathe mindfully. We may pause at the door and breathe mindfully every time we enter the room of a patient. We may use hand washing as a cue to breathe mindfully and then hold an intention for being present with our next patient or the patient's family.

We may use hand washing as a cue to breathe mindfully and then hold an intention for being present with our next patient or the patient's family.

The principle is simple: in mindfulness we direct our attention to our attention.

Where attention goes, neurons fire. And where neurons fire, our brains can rewire. In mindful awareness, we are stimulating neuronal activation and growth in our middle prefrontal regions. This kind of activity has the power to change us at a very deep level. Nhat Hanh guides us to pay attention to our breath as the trigger for directing our attention. He says, " . . . conscious breathing is an important bridge . . . by concentrating on our breathing 'in' and 'out,' we bring body and mind back together and become whole" (p. 12).

Three exercises for "in the moment" mindful practices are adapted from the work of Thich Nhat Hanh, and described below:

1. **Mindful breathing.** Begin with a refrain such as *Breathe in and know that I am breathing in; breathe out and know that I am breathing out.* When we are in touch with our breath, we are in touch with the simple miracle of being alive. We can tune in to our breath at any moment throughout the day, and when we do, we are present. Breath is always with us.

2. **Smiling.** You can begin every day with a smile. When we lose our smile (and there are plenty of reasons to

lose it in any given day) we simply breathe until we can regain it. A smile affirms our intention and awareness to live and work peacefully and compassionately. A smile helps us connect with our innate gentleness, and that gentleness reaches those around us.

3. **Body awareness and releasing tension.** Repeat the refrain: *Breathing in, I am aware of my body. Breathing out, I release the tension in my body.* An important practice is being aware of the tension we hold in our body, noticing and listening to what our body is telling us about itself. When we practice this awareness, we are more able to consciously release the tension through tuning in to our breath.

These exercises can be practiced throughout the day: while we are driving to work, while we are walking down the hallway, while we are preparing for a patient procedure or encounter, when we sit down to enter information into the computer. It is almost always possible to consciously breathe, smile, and release tension through mindful breathing. It is simple to incorporate these mindful habits into our daily routines, and as we integrate these practices we are training our minds and bodies—and metaphorically, our hearts—to be more aware, attuned, and present.

Summary of Key Thoughts

- Presence, all by itself, is healing.

- Our capacity for presence and attunement is shaped by our own early experiences, the belief systems that arose as a result of them, how we define ourselves as people, how we define our role as caregivers, and our conscious decisions.

- Attunement with another human being is one of our earliest quests. It seems likely that evolution is at the heart of it; we connect with each other in the beginning as part of a biological imperative to survive.

- The experience of the patient, who is often momentarily regressed, fearful, away from familiar and reassuring elements of his own environment, may be remarkably like the experience of the infant: searching, wondering about safety, needful of touch, needful of reassurance, needful of information about the environment, needful of one who is present and seeks to understand.

- As we develop into adults, we learn to cope with a lack of affect or a mis-attuned affect in others, but we never get comfortable with it. It doesn't feel good to encounter it, and it doesn't feel good to offer it to others.

- Attunement supports patients' self-regulation, the gathering of reliable information, and collaborative relationships between clinicians and patients/families.

- Co-regulation supports patients' self-regulation and their ability to physically and neurologically aid in their own healing. The scattered, distracted patient can become the calm, focused patient through co-regulation.

- The energy in the room changes when you enter it. Attunement allows us to more fully perceive the impact that our own presence in the room, the procedures we carry out, and our own movements and facial expressions have on the other.

- With your presence, with your eyes, with questions that are based on things that are meaningful to the patient, and perhaps with your touch, you find a way to connect. Presence, attunement, and co-regulation are achieved, if only for a moment or two.

- Attunement may take the mildest of adjustments: just remember to stop, touch the door jamb before you enter the room, breathe, count to five, and get ready to greet and intentionally attune to another human being.

- Siegel refers to reflection as the "fourth 'R' of education"; without reflection, part of our brain goes unused. Reflection develops the prefrontal cortex of the brain, which Siegel refers to as the neural hub of our humanity.

- Once we have consciously directed our attention to notice body movement, facial expression, changes in muscle tone or respiration, and other expressions of a person's state of being, we can reflect on how to use this information to attune.

- Attunement makes us curious about people; it inspires us to look with deep interest at another, to wonder.

- Attunement draws us into rhythmic interaction—a kind of reciprocal exchange—with another person.

- Attunement causes us to align ourselves with others, which may be evident in everything from our respiration to the next question we ask.

- Attunement means we see a person as a person, rather than as an obstacle or an object or a labeled category.

- Attunement means we have a stake in the welfare of the person to whom we are attuned.

- It is possible to breathe, smile, and release tension through mindful breathing.

Reflection

- Do you remember what it was like for someone to focus all of his or her attention on you and to occupy himself or herself with nothing more than attuning to you if only for a few seconds? Who was that person? What did that feel like to you?

- Consider specific times in your life, either personally or professionally, when you have been attuned to another. What was the result of those encounters for you and the other person? What conditions supported your being fully present?

- Consider specific times in your life, either personally or professionally, when you have been mis-attuned to another. What was the result of those encounters for you or the other person? What conditions contributed to your inability to be fully present?

- Make particular note of the energy states and behaviors of people in your care. In what way does their energy and behavior affect your ability to connect with them? What makes it most difficult for you to remain open and present?

- Time pressures often diminish our capacity to be aware and present. What are the ways in which time affects you? What are some ways in which you have successfully worked with time pressures and multiple priorities? What are some strategies for coping more effectively with time pressures and priorities in order to remain emotionally present with your patients?

• Identify one or two actions that you will incorporate into your practice in the next six weeks that will help you strengthen your ability to be present and attuned.

• Listen to "Just Two Words" and "My Caregiver's Stance for Today" from the *See Me as a Person* CD with a group of colleagues, and reflect together on what these passages mean to you and whether they inspire any changes in your practice.

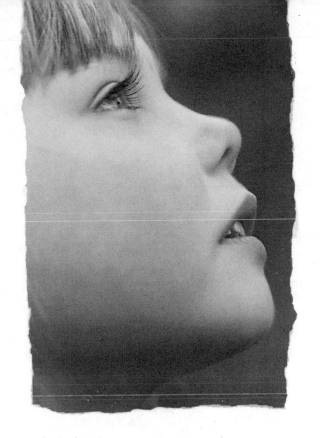

Chapter Three

Wondering:

Cultivating Curiosity for Efficient and Compassionate Practice

If we wonder often, the gift of knowledge will come.

—Native American Proverb

A new mother tells the pediatrician, "He won't eat." Indeed it appears to be so as James has dropped to the 3rd percentile in weight and is visibly smaller and less robust than when last examined. The mother, Sarah, talks at length, clearly distressed about many things at once: how her boyfriend left her, how the baby cries too much, and, and, and . . . . But the physician is distracted by the way Sarah is holding and feeding James even as she speaks. This six-month-old is facing out into the room, away from his mother, while she reaches around from behind his head to insert the rubber nipple into his mouth. There is no eye contact, no cuddling, no engagement that would allow this baby to soothe, settle, and take in some nourishment.

Based on her knowledge of infant feeding, the physician wonders if Sarah's feeding style could be contributing to the problem. If she could hold James with a little more closeness maybe this irritable, skinny baby could eat.

This is excellent wondering. And that wondering, so far, has given us a paradigm for understanding the baby's failure to gain weight that could save us a good deal of trouble and a good deal of money by making our clinical intervention match the actual problem, instead of delivering a batch of services to the baby that are actually off the mark.

Still, one more step in wondering is needed as the clinician develops the treatment plan. If the mother's feeding style is out of synch with the baby's developmental needs for touch, neurological regulation, and attachment, further wondering would lead to a heretofore unconsidered question: Why is Sarah feeding this way? Does she truly not know better? Does she think this is the optimal feeding style and merely needs redirection and education?

But the clinician has stopped wondering. It seems clear: Sarah doesn't know how to feed her baby. Somebody should teach her. So the clinician turns to didactics. She gives advice. Believing that Sarah must be ignorant on the matter, the doctor shows her a better way to hold her child.

Sarah nods. The wise pediatrician detects, even in that moment, that not a word of what she just said has gotten in, and she suspects that Sarah will likely not change her feeding methods.

Initially, the doctor did some pretty good wondering, didn't she? Her wondering evoked an idea, didn't it? She then competently conveyed her idea to Sarah, didn't she? Hadn't she handed her a plate of easily digestible information? All Sarah had to do was pick it up and take it in (sort of like the baby).

A true commitment to wondering makes a slightly greater demand on us. The version of wondering that the physician practiced served the needs of the clinician to find a solution or at least a solid theory about what the problem was. It was a good start, but it was only a start. She forgot to continue to be purposefully ignorant, naïve, open, curious, and ready to learn. Her wondering, and the paradigm that resulted from it, made the physician feel better. She was able to discern and then implement a solution to the problem that logically should have fixed it, but the solution did not produce the desired result. She stopped wondering too soon, thereby short-circuiting her own openness, her own curiosity, her own readiness to learn.

It would have taken only a little bit more devotion to the principle that the patient always has something to teach us. Without the patient's teaching we cannot really do our jobs. What was it that Sarah had been talking about just moments ago? Oh, yes. Boyfriend just left. But what could that have to do with an infant falling off the bottom of a growth chart?

Fortunately for us, we don't have to know the answer to that question. We just have to wonder about it. If we really believe that patients have things to teach us about their illness, then we become seriously devoted to listening to them, and this mother had something to say.

Sarah had named James after his father. When he walked out on her, what she believed to be true about herself was proven correct: she is unlovable, at least by males. Sarah expected to be left by males, and it just came true again. Now here she is, stuck and alone with a little baby—a boy, to boot. This one will leave her too after he no longer wants anything from her.

That, it turns out, is the answer to the question the doctor forgot to ask. Why is Sarah feeding in such an absurdly non-nurturing way? She's got James in a high chair, facing out into a very large, noisy room, while she stands at the kitchen counter, reaching around from behind the high chair to stick a bottle into his mouth. James is getting milk, more or less, but not nourishment. Sarah was in despair, and soon James would be too.

The pediatrician was actually right. This is why James was losing weight. She just needed to continue wondering just a little longer. If the pediatrician had not launched into education quite yet or if she had begun education but then stopped to ask questions as soon as she noticed that her efforts were being tuned out, she might have remembered something Sarah already taught her about the conditions under which she was caring for this baby. Then she could have asked the key question: "What has it been like for you since your boyfriend left?"

It happened that this pediatric practice sponsored a mothers' support group. There were lots of teen moms in this little village next to a big Air Force base, and the mothers' support group seemed to be an effective way to reduce maternal isolation, to give out information, and to keep track of the moms' progress. One day, not long after her visit with Sarah, the physician attended a meeting of the group. She sat with rapt attention as the other mothers asked Sarah how James was doing. It surprised her when Sarah told the truth: James was not doing well at all, and she was worried. ("She was?" the physician thought. "Then why wasn't she following the plan?") But the bigger surprise came when she watched Sarah's comrades come to her rescue. The other mothers didn't give advice about feeding practices. They simply commiserated with her. They asked about her life, learned that she had been abandoned, and they wondered how she had been feeling since James, Sr. took off. They shared stories of betrayal and loss. They showed empathy.

James started gaining weight in the following weeks. The physician was staggered to see why: Sarah was now holding him in a cradled position, looking directly into his eyes, and talking soothingly to him while she held his bottle. James was eagerly taking in the contents of his bottle, but he was also getting nourishment from his mother.

This intelligent, compassionate, experienced physician had been right all along. She only dropped the ball by moving away from the act of wondering—something that on some level she'd even begun adopting as a core practice—too quickly; she thought she had wondered enough, so she moved on to intervention. When the intervention didn't work, she blamed the mom who wasn't listening and wasn't changing.

What Sarah's comrades did for her was to wonder with her just a little bit more...

What Sarah's comrades did for her was to wonder with her just a little bit more. When Sarah got to say out loud how lost and distressed she was and how little confidence she had that her baby would love her back (after all, he was just another betraying male, wasn't he?), she began to release, to stop blaming baby James, to stop avoiding intimate contact with her own son. Sarah picked James up and resumed parenting him like a mom who really wanted him to eat and to thrive.

Health care, it turns out, is full of mysteries. In our efforts to eliminate the mysteries, to conquer disease, to heal our fellow beings, surely we cannot forget the most basic tool we have: the capacity to look and really see, to ask and really listen, to wonder and really discover.

Wondering is a courageous act—an extension of attention and focus on behalf of another.

On Becoming Empty

"Becoming empty" may sound like a terrifying prospect for a health care professional. Aren't we being paid to know? Don't patients demand that? Indeed, we seem to be subject to a particular—perhaps even contractual—division of labor: You (the patient) will present a problem to me. I (the health care provider) will tell you what it is and how to fix it.

There are two problems with getting too carried away with these presumptions. First, we can become anti-scientific. We may conclude too early and then close down our wondering minds. No more data get in. We may be unwilling to change our minds (or even reopen them), so we overlook things and we make mistakes.

Second, we can become disinterested in the person—or at least the fullest self of the person. We focus on the problem as we have defined it and lose our ability to wonder about the rest of the person: what this illness means to her or her family, what other things he is saying about the symptoms that we have overlooked or ignored because it didn't fit with our conclusions about the problem, what the treatment we have proposed means to him or his family (and therefore whether the patient and family are likely to follow through with treatment).

Wondering is a step on the path to becoming mindful, which is increasingly understood as key to discovering new things about ourselves and our patients. Mindful learning can be characterized by "intelligent ignorance, flexible thinking, the avoidance of premature cognitive commitments, and creative uncertainty" (Siegel, 2007, p. 234). A platform for the sort of scientific inquiry that becomes possible through mindfulness was suggested by Langer (1997, p. 111, formatting ours):

When we are mindful, we implicitly or explicitly do the following:

1. We view a situation from several perspectives.

2. We see information presented in the situation as novel.

3. We attend to the context in which we are perceiving the information.

4. We create new categories through which this information may be understood.

These decidedly anti-conclusive qualities and practices constitute the core of wondering. Wondering allows us to *not know* on purpose because it turns out that we are better learners when our minds are still a little uncertain and therefore still open.

Wondering allows us to be brilliantly stupid—having decided, as a result of all of our knowledge, to set aside our presumptions and open ourselves to the data in front of us, the data that only emerge when we ask and when we wonder. Wondering allows us to have an elite athlete's mind: loose, flexible, ready to change course, ready to try on new possibilities. Wondering allows us to go slowly toward locking down our theories about the patient and perhaps to remain reverent enough not to.

The patient who shows up on the anniversary of her husband's death, year after year, always complaining of the same symptoms, deserves a clinician who will set aside his technology, who will set aside his considerable wisdom and experience with the nuances of her symptoms, and just wonder with her. It does not take more time. It may, in fact, be quite a cost savings to nip this anniversary-specific exacerbation of symptoms in the bud by just wondering: "Stella, it's April again. I've noticed that you always come to see me in the spring. It just dawned on me that this is around the same the time of year when Howard died. Can we talk about whether there could be any connection between your symptoms getting worse in the spring, and the passing of your beloved Howard?"

Wondering allows you to reorient yourself to the place from which wisdom comes. It doesn't come from what you already know; it comes from discovering what you don't know.

Humility as a Prerequisite for Wondering

Take a moment to ask yourself this question: If one of the people you cherish most in this world was about to have major surgery, would you want the surgeon to be confident? Would you want the nurses caring for your loved one to be confident? We imagine that you would.

Now consider this question: Would you want your loved one's surgeon and nurses to be humble?

This, we imagine, is a more complex question—and one that requires a more reflective explanation. It requires consideration of exactly what it means to be humble. Jayne Felgen (2004) opens up the meaning of humility by comparing one's entrance into the patient's world to a border crossing.

When a care provider crosses the threshold of a patient and family's door, he or she crosses a border, moving from the world of practical preparation into that of a personal healing relationship in which everything he or she does is in service to the patient. This border crossing brings care providers into the patient's and family's world—a world about which they know little—and within which they must tread with great humility. (p. 23)

Felgen's words invite us to look at humility with new eyes. Perhaps we can dismiss our preconceived notions about humility, beginning with its semantic relationship with the word *humiliation*.

Humility is commonly defined as "having a modest opinion or estimate of one's own importance, rank, status, etc. . . . or, the quality of not thinking you are better than other people." The idea of "treading with great humility" when we care for patients is a counterintuitive notion for some of us who have been acculturated to believe that clinical excellence in today's fast-paced health care environments draws on a very different set of human characteristics. It's possible that it even runs counter to our core sense of responsibility to guide and protect our patients.

In philosophy texts going back as far as Socrates, epistemic humility is defined as knowing that we as mere human beings have limits to our knowledge, and that wisdom comes from realizing that we cannot know all that we need to know in order to draw meaningful conclusions about people. Instead, humility puts us in the position to wonder about the person we're caring for as a fundamental condition for good care.

A physician colleague told us about a significant teacher in his past who cautioned him against assuming that any diagnosis is final. His teacher said, "When a 'final' diagnosis is made, you quit thinking about what else may be causing the problem, and you quit listening to your patient. Every diagnosis should be a 'working' diagnosis, always susceptible to change with new information." This is a humble position from which to work, and it's one that serves patients well.

In medicine there's so much mystery even in what we think we know conclusively about our patients. An X-ray can conclusively detect a broken bone, but it can tell us next to nothing about the person who will be going through the experience of that bone's healing. Two people of roughly the same age are given what appears to be the same cancer diagnosis at the same time; one lives for two months while the other lives for five years. What makes the difference in these instances, and what of that difference can be known conclusively at any point?

In health care, living in the eternal mystery of what we don't know must go hand-in-hand with anything we think we do know. Carl Jung speaks to his own struggle with this very real paradox in this excerpt from his 1957 work, *The Undiscovered Self*:

> If I want to understand an individual human being, I must lay aside all scientific knowledge of the average man and discard all theories in order to adopt a completely new and unprejudiced attitude. I can only approach the task of understanding with a free and open mind, whereas knowledge of persons, or insight into human character, presupposes all sorts of knowledge about mankind in general. Now, whether it is a question of understanding a fellow human being or of self-knowledge, I must in both cases leave all theoretical assumptions behind me. (p. 9)

As clinicians we are constantly balancing scientific knowledge with understanding the individual before us. There is mystery in even the most straightforward diagnosis because there is complexity and mystery in every human being. No matter what you believe about the mind-body connection, few dispute any longer that the state of a person's mind affects his or her healing process. The mind that buys into the prognosis of "two months to live" is far more likely to fulfill that prophesy than is the mind that embraces the infinite mystery of the human body's well-proven ability to self-correct under the right conditions.

If we bring humility to practice, we're open to observing infinitely more about each unique condition being experienced by each unique patient. When we bring humility, we can remain curious and continue to learn.

Humble clinicians know what they know and are equally aware of what they don't know. There is no threat in not knowing everything—in fact, there is wisdom in understanding that truth. Humility leads to a thoughtful and thorough assessment in partnership with the patient and family.

Few would argue that it's the height of arrogance to think that one knows everything. But we'd like to suggest that it takes no small measure of arrogance to think that one knows much of anything about a human being with whom he or she has not yet spent any time in relationship. With humility we can ask our patients, "What's most important to you today?" and accept that anything the patient sees as important is important because it provides us with information about what he needs and perhaps some small insight into who he is. A therapeutic interchange is fundamental to gaining the knowledge essential to care, and greater understanding of the patient as a person is the primary goal. If you often use questions and phrases such as the following when interacting with patients, then you are probably exercising humility:

- "Please tell me what you meant by_____."

- "Is there something more that I need to know about this?"

- "What is most important to you?"

- "I'm not sure I know what that word means."

- "Would you explain this to me?"

- "I notice that _____; does that seem accurate to you?"

- "What, if anything, worries you now?"

Humility is most likely to be a characteristic of those care-givers who are grounded and proficient in their clinical art and craft and who have developed the capacity to "get themselves out of the way" and be truly interested in both their patients and their colleagues. We are socialized into our professional roles with a spoken or unspoken expectation that we are knowledgeable experts. Our challenge is to accept the respon-sibility inherent in this role expectation while developing the commensurate humility that allows us to remain open, to learn, and to deepen our understanding of the complexity and mystery of human caring.

Humility begins with unconditional acceptance of what is most human in us. It means to accept that we, like all other human beings, do not need to be perfect. With this acceptance of our beauty and our ugliness, our suffering and our resil-ience, the divide between ourselves and others is diminished and we experience the grace of human connection. True rela-tionship requires humility. We must be open and accessible to others if we are to know them and allow them to know us.

Wondering: What it Is, and What it Isn't

Wondering is Noticing and Inquiring, Not Interrogating and Collecting Data

The electronic health record (EHR) is a tremendous asset and advancement in our ability to provide coordinated and comprehensive care. It's been proven to improve legibility of clinical records, reduce prescription errors, enhance access to guidelines and best practices, support patients' access to their own information, and facilitate communication and exchange of information among health care professionals and hospitals and clinics. This advancement in technology is not only highly valuable to the clinician in describing, communicating, and monitoring care; it is becoming increasingly valuable to people receiving care, as their history is at the fingertips of their caregivers. Clearly, the EHR enhances the provision of safe care.

The potential dark side of such an advancement in technology, however, is that unless it is perceived as a tool and not the driver of care, it will absolutely interfere with the clinician-patient relationship and compromise the accuracy of the assessment (Barager, April 2011).

Such interference occurred for a mother who took her adolescent daughter into the emergency department as directed by the clinic physician who first saw the child. The daughter was experiencing extreme abdominal pain and had a history of chronic illness that made her symptoms very concerning to the physician and the mother. Upon their arrival in the ER, the triage nurse conducted an intake assessment. The assessment consisted of a list of standardized questions on a computer screen, and the mother grew increasingly agitated as the nurse kept her attention fixed squarely on her computer screen rather than on the girl writhing in pain in front of her. The nurse did not look at the girl; she did not comment on her discomfort, and in fact she seemed to not even notice it. Instead, she efficiently went about her business of collecting information. At the end of the data collection, she politely told the mother and daughter to have a seat in the waiting room. The ER physician would be able to see them in approximately 90 minutes.

The mother was shocked and asked if there was something that could be done sooner. She clarified that she had in fact called ahead and that the physician in the clinic told them to come right in, which they did without delay. She also pointed out, though it felt ludicrous to do so once again, that her daughter was clearly in severe pain. The nurse responded that the physician was busy with other patients and would not able to see her for 90 minutes; further, the nurse could not do anything for the pain, she said, until the girl was seen by a physician. The mother was upset and went to the front desk, asked for a phone, called the other emergency department in the same city, and took her daughter there.

In contrast, the triage nurse in the other emergency department started by assessing the physical status of the daughter and inquiring about why the mother thought this was happening and what she needed to know in order to take care of the child. She helped the girl lie down on a stretcher, positioned her to ease her pain, and began a thorough physical assessment. The daughter began to calm down immediately due to the attentive ministrations of the triage nurse.

We need to be conscious of the way we are integrating information systems into our practice.

The first scenario demonstrates an extreme example of failing to wonder—of seeing the intake assessment as a process of collecting information rather than learning about the person. We need to be conscious of the way we are integrating information systems into our practice. Does the computer screen expand our capacity to take in information or does it inhibit our ability to use all of our senses to observe and notice as we are learning about the person needing care? While the difference between these two experiences may have something to do with the two different hospital cultures, there is much that you as an individual clinician can do to make a difference. In the second hospital, the triage nurse would have to fill out the same paperwork as the nurse at the first hospital. She made the decision, however, to see the patient as a person, and to put the person ahead of the protocol. For more information on how to remain present with our patients despite our professional obligation to observe protocols, please see Appendix B on page 390.

Wondering is Accepting, not Judging

Some patients have personalities only a mother can love! That is a fact of life. As clinicians we are called upon to be conscious of our own biases and our human tendency to discount or judge. We may be predisposed to judge by our own histories, experiences, and triggers, and even by the caregiver who preceded us, who may have relayed information that labeled or categorized the person in our care in some way. Accepting another person without judgment is a mindful and conscious act. One of Mary's teachers counseled novice clinicians to "scan for biases" before they entered a room. This guidance resonated with many of the students, and they seemed able to consciously translate this into their practice.

In health care it's inevitable that we cross paths with much that is unsavory. Throughout the course of our work, all five senses are challenged and sometimes even assaulted. The following story, told by a health care provider in one of our workshops, illustrates this perfectly:

"You're Not Cut Out for Nursing"

When I was 15 years old, I visited my grandmother in a nursing home and told her that I wanted to be a nurse. My grandmother had been a nurse for many decades, and because I admired my grandmother more than anyone else, I wanted to follow in her footsteps.

I was surprised at her reaction as she immediately told me that I was not cut out for nursing. Seeing that I was all but crushed, she said, "Come back tomorrow and ask to see Mr.

Perkins. He's a resident here; he likes to play cards. You play cards with him tomorrow and then tell me about your experience."

The next day I came to the nursing home and spent an hour playing cards with Mr. Perkins. I then visited my grandmother who asked me about the experience. I told her the truth—that I had loved getting to know Mr. Perkins, that he made me laugh, had a lot of stories to share, and was a great card player. I told her that we'd made a date for me to return in a few days.

What I didn't mention was that Mr. Perkins was severely disfigured.

My grandmother pulled me close in a tight, loving hug and told me that I would in fact make a very good nurse.

Wondering is Discovering, not Assuming

A pediatric nurse practitioner described seeing a toddler in the clinic who presented with a fever and history of ear infections. He was crying and flailing and needed immediate attention to ease the pain and treat the infection. It took a while to help him calm down. Once the child quieted, the practitioner turned her attention to the rest of the family and noticed the mother sitting to the side with her two small daughters. She remembers the encounter this way:

Something Seemed Off

I couldn't figure out what it was, but something seemed off. I noticed that both girls were still dressed in their pajamas and bunny slippers and it was midday. I said, "I notice the girls are still in their pajamas." The mother looked straight at me and said, "Yes, that's why we're here." ("Not for your son's ear infection?" I thought the question but kept silent.) She began to cry and said, "My father is abusing them as he did me and my sister. We never told anyone."

I was stunned. There is no way I was expecting that, and if I had not taken the moment to pay attention to my inner sense of unease and to put words to what I noticed, I don't know if the mother would have said anything. It was only a moment, and it could easily have been lost.

This case description points out several concrete aspects of wondering:

- The nurse practitioner paused and noticed; she used her eyes.

- She tuned into, and did not dismiss, her sense of unease, which happens when we pay attention to the subtle clues in assessment including our "gut feelings."

- She put her wondering into words and was open to hearing the response no matter what that response might be.

Wondering is Staying Open, not Rushing to Conclusions

A few years ago, Michael described persistent jaw pain to his internist during a routine exam. No serious inquiry was conducted. The physician concluded that this was a dental issue, since it occurred in his mouth. A referral was made, and the dentist concurred that there was a dental issue. (Remember the old adage: "To the hammer, everything looks like a nail"?) He referred Michael on to an oral surgeon who prescribed a root canal. There were problems with the first procedure, so it had to be repeated—twice. The pain remained. Time passed.

Mary, however, continued to wonder, which was perfectly natural because she had unlimited time for Michael, and as he is someone about whom she cares deeply, she could not help but see him as a whole person.

In spite of the medical history which indicated that Michael's father had multiple heart attacks at a younger age than Michael was now, the clinicians had not considered his heart as a possible source of the pain. But Mary looked up "jaw pain," and it was right there: jaw pain can be angina. A stress test was requested, and Michael flunked it. Further tests revealed the possibility of a heart issue so an angioplasty was scheduled. This procedure was interrupted by the surprising discovery of more than 90% blockage in four arteries. A bypass was scheduled for the next morning.

Michael didn't die, of course, and he even managed to side-step a heart attack, but a year had passed since he first described the jaw pain, and much money, time, and discomfort was poured into the hole while we chased, with too much certainty and too little wondering, a premature conclusion.

What would have happened if anyone along the way—the internist, the nurse in that office, the dentist, the oral surgeon, anyone we stumbled across during that strange year—had come to Michael with an empty mind? What would have happened if any one of the clinicians had wondered beyond what appeared to be obvious?

At the very least, the camera that had too quickly become focused on Michael's mouth would have backed up and seen him as a whole person. What is in his health history that could have given a clue? Perhaps only a clinician dedicated to discovery, rather than to fixing the first thing that appeared to be broken, would have been inclined to look in the chart and notice the paternal medical history. The lens needed to be wider.

Had anyone wondered just a bit longer, this year-long delay, which increased the risk that he might suffer a massive heart attack, might have been avoided. He would have felt seen. Medical mistakes would have been avoided. We would have saved a few thousand dollars spent on root canals and cleared the chair for people who really needed those services. The system of scientific inquiry, consideration, and development of a working hypothesis that is supposed to characterize health care, but can happen only if we start with an empty mind, would have worked.

Wondering is Remembering that Everybody has a Back Story

This is extremely important. In fast-paced health care settings, we may never know a person's back story. Simply remembering that we all have a back story helps us to stay open, accepting, and clear that there is always more to be learned and much that we will never know.

For instance, a clinician once told us about an ethics consult that was requested for a woman on public assistance who had been in the intensive care unit for months. She suffered from a systemic, necrotizing soft tissue infection complicated by a history of drug abuse, malnutrition, and a combination of other disease factors. She was barely surviving, and experiencing great pain and suffering. Her prognosis was dire; she was not going to survive, yet she was insistent that the team continue aggressive measures to prolong her life as long as possible. In the process of the ethics inquiry the hospital pastor discovered that the woman had lived as a prostitute, and the reason she could not let go and allow death was her terror that she was condemned to hell because of her life on earth. Despite all of her physical pain, spiritual care was her greatest need.

In another case, a clinician puzzled over a 395-pound man undergoing bariatric surgery. He was not easy to connect with, was easily agitated, and seemed bossy. The clinician knew that people who are morbidly obese and choose elective bariatric surgery can be subject to disapproval, judgment, and stereotyping, and she acknowledged this as an area of potential bias. She later learned that this man was grieving the murder of his adolescent daughter. Since her devastating death, he literally tried to eat himself to death. This elective surgery was his first step toward choosing life.

We may never know the story, but when we wonder, we will simply remember that there is one. When we remember, our attitude and behaviors change.

Wondering is a philosophical and practical practice that helps us to avoid our tendency to judge and even condemn another. Wondering about the back story puts us in a position to connect and learn, whether we ever actually learn the back story or not.

What Happens When We Forget to Wonder?

It happens to us sometimes: we forget to be curious about our patients. Sometimes it's purposeful; we think we don't have time. Sometimes we are unconscious of our absence of wonder, never catching on until the patient goes home—or just goes away. Sometimes we never do come to understand what our simple inability to wonder—to walk into the room purposefully ignorant, naïve, open, curious, ready to learn—has meant to the diagnosis (where we may miss something crucially important), to the treatment (where we apply perfectly good methods to an illness we do not fully understand, at least as it manifests in this patient) or to aftercare (where the insulted, ignored, or simply not-fully-understood patient regains his power and now ignores us).

In the remarkable 2009 film *Mother and Child*, Elizabeth, relinquished for adoption by her 14-year-old birth mother, grows into a dynamic, beautiful, intelligent woman who avoids intimacy like the plague. She'd gone to Mexico for a tubal ligation as a 17-year-old—an historical fact learned by her physician many years later when she went in to discover why she was showing signs of pregnancy. By then she was a successful, driven lawyer. Since she had just revealed that she'd taken measures long ago to ensure that she'd never get pregnant, surely the doctor can be forgiven for assuming that the news that she is now pregnant will not be welcomed by her patient.

The problem is that it seems to never occur to the physician—portrayed in the film as kind, competent, concerned, not devoid of empathy—to wonder what this mid-30s adoptee might actually want. After all, her patient once went to a great deal of trouble to prevent pregnancy. She's single; she certainly doesn't seem very maternal (whatever that means) nor ready to rearrange her busy life to accommodate a child.

So we can hardly condemn the doctor for delivering the news that Elizabeth is pregnant and following it immediately with, "So you can talk to the staff up front about coming in, and we'll take care of it. Then we can talk about other forms of birth control. OK?"

The doctor departs. The whole interaction takes 30 seconds. The patient never speaks; she is never asked to speak. She sits, dumbfounded, for several seconds, then walks quietly out of the exam room to the reception desk where she does a clean and violent sweep of everything on the counter with one arm. Disturbed by the noise, the physician comes running out, where she is confronted by the patient: "You don't know who I am, or what I want, you @&%*!"

Elizabeth probably won't be coming back for prenatal care. Evidently she won't be making that appointment to "take care of it" either. She had something else in mind—although maybe even she didn't know what. After all, she had only a few seconds to digest this earth-shattering news and to put it together with the loss of her mother at birth and her long-held defenses against motherhood or any kind of human intimacy. Elizabeth might not have been particularly articulate or clear-headed even if the physician had bothered to inquire about her wishes or if a nurse had stopped in just to say, "Wow. Big news. How can we help?"

We didn't have to read her mind, though. We didn't have to do anything, really, except to make a tiny bit of space in our own minds to wonder about what pregnancy could mean to this person named Elizabeth at this particular time in her life with the particular experiences that had been hers in that life. We didn't have to know the answer in order for this to come out better for everyone involved. We just had to wonder.

It can be a terrifying thing, really. People come to us for answers. Indeed, they come to us demanding answers and they're sometimes not very nice about it. We carry the mantle of expertise, and this suggests that something directive, or scientific, or at least smart ought to come out of our mouths when we put on the mantle. Can we really presume to call it *medicine* or *nursing* or even *practice* in those moments in which we bring only curiosity to the table?

Trading even one drop of presumption for a moment of pure curiosity opens us to operate with limitless data at our fingertips.

We can and must, because curiosity—the suspension of every bit of our presumption that we already know what's going on in front of us—helps us to do everything else better. Trading even one drop of presumption for a moment of pure curiosity opens us to operate with limitless data at our fingertips. In a moment of curiosity, we are empathetic and connected. As new, unexpected information and understanding surface, we cannot help but operate with greater precision.

The 15-year-old lupus patient wouldn't seem to be an expert on much (except worrying her parents), but she does know this: after a gazillion sticks in the two years since she got sick, she knows where the nurse or the tech is most likely to be successful with the blood draw. Yet she is astonished to notice that they don't ask, and more often than not, they take offense when she tries to tell them. Persistently, they forget to wonder, even when it would make their jobs far easier.

They could be more efficient, they would have more time for other patients, and they could have more fun with this irritable adolescent. She thinks some of them act as if they have something to prove, like the nurse who said to her, "I've been doing this for nine years. I know how to find a vein"—and then missed, then went to find a supervisor—rather than just wonder and then ask this patient what her experience is with her own body.

Why is Wondering Often Difficult?

For neurological and cultural reasons, or because of our professional training, it may be inevitable that we become poor wonderers. Siegel (2007) points out:

> The brain has a natural drive to detect patterns. As an associational organ, it clusters those patterns into mental models that automatically classify the world into generalized schema that help us to rapidly sort through the huge amount of data in present sensation and in memory. (p. 251)

It's what we were trained to do: notice patterns, detect categories, and respond accordingly. There's nothing here, however, that suggests that the brain goes looking for additional information. Instead it goes directly to the work of clustering and classifying what is already known.

This would suggest that unless you train your brain to wonder, it doesn't.

Indeed, neurologist Antonio Damasio, head of the Neurology Department at the University of Iowa College of Medicine, suggests that such automatic categorizing and distilling is an essential aspect of learning, problem solving, and daily mental functioning. His *somatic marker hypothesis* (2003) posits that even before we think about something, a sort of automatic response to it begins to form, based on our real or perceived prior experience with that problem or experience. The hypothesis suggests that we save ourselves huge amounts of mental energy through this process, which really begins with a "gut feeling" (somatic marker). He proposes that this gut feeling sets off a process which causes us to engage in a sort of near-automatic decision-tree analysis.

The suggestion is that nurses, physicians, and other health care professionals (as well as everybody else on the planet) engage in this sort of decision making all day long. If we reject tried and true hypotheses and open ourselves to novelty, we subconsciously fear that everything will come to a screeching halt.

The proposition that wondering has a noble, practical, and respectable place in daily practice—yes, even in fast-paced clinical settings—is based on the discovery that reliance on categorical thinking can lead to "premature *hardening of the categories* [emphasis added], shutting down learning, and seeing . . . through old lenses" (Siegel, 2007, p. 252).

Wondering goes against the grain. It threatens our hard-won ways of knowing. It challenges us to be present, and it makes this patient, at this moment, under these circumstances, appear to us as a brand-new scientific challenge filled with novelty, rife with all of the awe-inspiring complexity of personhood.

For example, let's say we encounter an angry person in the hallway. What happens first? Damasio would propose that even before we are able to collect all the data about the event and develop a detailed, rational plan for responding, a somatic marker erupts: "Whoa. I've been here before. I need to get this under control."

The somatic marker may reflect an experience we had with a bully when we were in the third grade, or a time when we were flooded with our own rage, or even a lesson learned from an honored professor in nursing or medical school. It tells us the category (perhaps "nutcase" or "interruption of routine" or "could lead to violence"), and perhaps most unfortunately, it leads us to conclusions based on prior information rather than prompting us to collect new information that may have something to do with what's actually going on in front of us.

Our very wiring encourages us to shut ourselves off from the real person being angry and to develop a response principally based on our earlier experience with "people like this" or "this sort of thing." Our response becomes strangely impersonal, unrelated to the person in front of us; creative problem-solving goes out the window just when we need it most. Not surprisingly, this inadvertent dismissiveness toward the person in front of us tends to exacerbate the situation. The patient becomes angrier because he is not seen. He knows he is being managed, not responded to authentically. He may walk away and later take it out on the hospital or us. Or he may yell louder, trying to get what he wants most: our genuine attention, our empathy, our help.

But what would our practice be like, if in the face of patient or family anger, our first impulse was to wonder? What if we could question the knee-jerk conclusions of the somatic marker, soften the categories, and return to being a compassionate scientist who is always dedicated to understanding what is right in front of us without presumptions and just wondering?

What would our practice be like, if in the face of patient or family anger, our first impulse was to wonder?

What if we imagined the distant possibility that the patient or family member actually has something to be angry about?

What if we wondered who or what the patient had been contending with before we came upon the scene? What if we entertained the notion that the patient's anger is a not-altogether-crazy response to his being sick, and to his being powerless over that sickness, and to his being further powerless over the institutions in which sick people often find themselves, and to his being further powerless to even get someone to come finish the admitting process so some care can be delivered, and to his being further powerless to get residents to stop trooping through, one after another, seeing his humiliatingly vulnerable and weak self lying there like a baby?

When all of that explodes in the clinician's face—the one who did nothing except step into the room—are you ready to be honestly curious about why? Might that indeed be a terrific time to also be curious about what this patient's condition might mean to him? Might the two minutes it would take to earnestly inquire constitute an investment that would save many minutes of time wasted in trying to calm him down or to stop him from hammering the call light or hiding his medications?

Among other things, wondering is the simple act of becoming informed. Becoming informed honors the informant, reduces the patient's resistance, and increases cooperation, and along the way, it changes the clinician. The act of wondering, the process of learning what needs to be known in order to deliver care to this particular patient, the attitude shift that accompanies the commitment to "intelligent ignorance, flexible thinking, the avoidance of premature cognitive commitments, and creative uncertainty" (Siegel, 2007, p. 234)—these things change us, and they don't just change us into nicer people; they change us into better scientists, better diagnosticians, and more effective clinicians.

Because your neurology actually works against your ability to wonder, it's extremely important to make the conscious choice to add a propensity for wonder into the way you practice every day. Your brain does not wonder on its own; it must be trained to do so. Fortunately, over time, neurology changes and those thoughts, deeds, and ways of being that you practice most will become your default way of being.

What Happens When We Commit to Curiosity?

Harvard psychiatry professor Arthur Kleinman proposes that there are novel ways to inquire about a patient's illness that significantly enhance our ability to obtain meaningful, relevant information in the health care interview. In his paradigm for inquiry, questions are better understood by the patient, answers are more complete, and hints are given about cultural, familial, or other factors that are likely to affect the ability of the patient to take in and retain information as well as the likelihood that the patient and family will follow through with aftercare. In effect, Kleinman's interview design suggests that we, the health care providers, need education about the family in order for efficacious care to be provided (Kleinman, Eisenburg, & Good, 1978).

His methods not only require an initial posture of wondering but also help us continue to wonder throughout care, no matter what we discover.

Kleinman outlines eight key questions in his work. We'll focus here only on the first question, but the complete list appears in Appendix C on page 395. He would have us begin by asking about the patient's or family member's perspective on the illness. What do they call it? Why do they believe the patient or family member is in the hospital?

Sometimes we are stopped short, right at the outset, with the discovery that our understanding about what is wrong and why the patient is here is markedly different from the patient's or family member's understanding. It is here that we may learn about family legends, tribal beliefs, religious overtones, themes of punishment for past sins, or connections with illnesses of other family members long ago. Remember the woman who had lived as a prostitute in the story on page 112? She had strong, fearful beliefs that were ultimately influencing her care. Providing her with the most efficacious care was difficult until we knew more about the contents of her mind and heart.

You might reasonably wonder why this sort of information would have any importance at all. If someone believes that she's ill because of a family curse, how could that possibly influence how we might care for her? And deep down, do we really want to know?

In instances like this one, it's likely that what stops our wondering most often is the fear that we won't be able to deal effectively with what we discover. If we're in our fix-it mode we want to be able to work efficiently with any information that comes to light, and sometimes what comes to light—for example, deep belief in superstitions, irrational fears, or soul-crushing guilt—is completely unscientific and well outside the realm of what we can fix.

Still, wouldn't we want to know if the patient believes his heart condition is an inevitable result of an affair he had three years ago, or that a spouse believes that the patient is not sick at all, but just malingering in order to avoid work? Wouldn't we want to know if the patient has given up based on a misunderstanding of something another health care provider said about the seriousness of his illness? These may be fixable conditions or they may not be, but it's all information that gives us insight into the patient and family.

Using wondering during intake, we would inquire about what the patient or family member believes about what caused the patient's problem. We've asked a factual question, and the scientist in us is hoping for a factual answer, but we're dealing with people, so it can't be counted on to go that way, and we may find ourselves invited into the patient's world of superstition, fear, guilt, or faulty cause-and-effect linking. The scientist in us may squirm just thinking about it, but the caregiver is intrigued.

"This patient is in my care," the clinician might think. "I want to learn all I need to know in order to provide her with the most efficient and effective care."

The caregiver in me wants to know if the patient believes the problem started with an infection caused by the IV used the last time he was in this very hospital. The caregiver in me wonders how this might impact his receptiveness to the IV someone is going to try to administer in just a few minutes. The caregiver in me wonders whether he may now be suspicious about other procedures done at this institution—or if he may even be suspicious of me. If this patient is in my care, all of this matters to me, because I am a caregiver.

Our patients come from everywhere. They've been to places we could never imagine. They've seen and done things that would turn us green with envy or give us nightmares for weeks. Until we begin to wonder about them, we don't know them at all.

Here are examples of 17 more things patients and families may be experiencing which we'll discover only if we wonder:

- The patient expects to die from her illness.

- The patient is ready to die.

- The patient is not ready to die.

- The patient has resigned himself to a life of chronic pain.

- The patient fears that she will be disfigured by her treatment and that her husband will leave her because of it.

- The patient believes that his illness has brought the family together, and his getting well will make the family fall apart again.

- Most of the patient's family members resent him because they told him to change his diet and he didn't; they blame him for his heart attack.

- The patient is fixated on her fear that no one will visit her while she is hospitalized and that the nurses will see that she is unloved.

- The patient's mother believes she will be ruined financially by this experience.

- The patient believes that the nurses will like her more if she "just goes without" instead of asking for what she wants.

- The patient intends to commit suicide.

- The patient has had terrible experiences with doctors.

- The patient's mother distrusts men.

- The patient is hoping his wife will come back to him because of his illness.

- The patient is acculturated to agree with anything a medical professional says, but has limited understanding of what's being said to him and no intention of following through.

- The patient is overly concerned with how you see her, so she's always cheerful and cooperative even though she's terrified.

- The patient is overwhelmed with shame every time he talks with his doctor because he has no insurance.

The patient's state of being is already in place whether it's secret from us or visible. As scientists and caregivers, we'd rather it was visible.

We invite you to check in with yourself at this point: Does this world of wondering feel to you like a Pandora's Box that you're reluctant to open because of the ever-tightening protocols that dictate how you spend your time? Or does it feel more like the very reason you went into health care?

The practice of wondering never stops. It does not have to create answers. Making it part of care right from the first appointment or admission means we might get to know our patient better, might be able to predict response to care better, might be able to head off problems through the course of the illness or treatment better, might be able to see patterns in the patient's illness and care history better, and might be able to understand the context of illness better for all our patients. Wondering promotes good science, good care, and good business.

Language for Wondering

Wondering language is open-ended and frequently includes "what" questions. It is grounded in true curiosity for what the other has to teach us. Some examples of wondering language (specifically, as it relates to humility) are provided on pages 104 and 105, and a more comprehensive selection of wondering language appears in the box on the following page.

Verbal Wondering Language
I wonder . . .
What is on the front of your mind right now?
What is most important to you?
I noticed that _____; does that seem accurate to you?
Would you explain this to me?
What do you think has caused your_____?
What do you most fear?
What worries you?
What do you think your illness means to your family?
Are you worried about anyone in your family?
What happened when _____?
How do you feel about _____?
In what way has this changed your life or the lives of your family?
What has been your past experience with _____? (e.g. IV start, care in a hospital, etc.)

Summary of Key Thoughts

- Wondering is an extension of attention and focus on behalf of another.

- Wondering is a philosophical and practical practice that helps us to avoid our tendency to judge and even condemn another. Wondering is a courageous act.

- Wondering is a step on the path to becoming mindful which is increasingly understood as key to discovering new data relative to ourselves and to our patients.

- Wondering is discovering, not assuming. Wondering allows us to be brilliantly stupid—choosing to set aside our presumptions and open ourselves to the data in front of us, the data that only emerge when we wonder.

- Wondering allows us to have an elite athlete's mind: loose, flexible, ready to change course, ready to try on new possibilities.

- Wondering is noticing and inquiring, not interrogating and collecting data.

- Clinicians must look up from the computer and see and listen to the person in their care. Technology is a tool. When technology is the driver of care, it interferes with the clinician-patient relationship and compromises the accuracy of the assessment.

- Wondering is accepting, not judging. Always "scan for biases" before entering a room.

- Wondering is staying open, not rushing to conclusions. The system of scientific inquiry, consideration, and development of a working hypothesis that is supposed to characterize health care can happen only if we start with an empty mind.

- Wondering is remembering that everybody has a back story. We may never know the back story, but when we wonder we will simply remember that there is one and that will affect the nature of our relationship.

- In a moment of curiosity, we are empathetic and connected. As new, unexpected information and understanding surfaces, we cannot help but operate with greater precision.

- Wondering is the simple act of becoming informed. Becoming informed honors the informant, reduces patient resistance, and increases cooperation. It also changes us as clinicians—and not just into being nicer people. We are changed into better scientists, better diagnosticians, and more effective caregivers.

- Wondering promotes good care, good science, and good business.

Reflection

- Consider this question: "Might the two minutes it would take to earnestly inquire about the condition of the patient-as-a-person constitute an investment that would save many minutes of time wasted in trying to calm him down or to stop him from being constantly on the call light, etc.?" What do you think about this? What meaning does it have for your practice? What meaning does it have for your work as a member of a health care team?

- Consider this question: "What if we imagined the possibility that the patient or family member actually has something to be angry about?" What memories does this question stir in you? Describe a case in which you recognized a patient or family member's anger as valid and legitimate. What happened? How did your recognition of the legitimacy of their anger affect your care?

- Clinicians have relayed the following concern about wondering: "It's likely that what stops my wondering most often is the fear that I won't be able to deal effectively with what I discover." What are your thoughts about this? What does it mean in your practice?

- What thoughts or beliefs might you need to change to improve your ability to wonder?

- Describe a time in your practice in which wondering resulted in learning about a back story or another discovery that made a difference for your patient's healing.

- Reflect on the meaning of humility in your practice. Think about humble clinicians you have worked with and how this quality affected their ability to wonder and relate to their patients and their colleagues. What did you notice? What was their impact?

- Pay attention to the moments when you're disturbed by someone's words or actions. What happens to your experience if you say to yourself, "I wonder what his back story is?"

- In what ways do you think wondering promotes good care, good science, and good business?

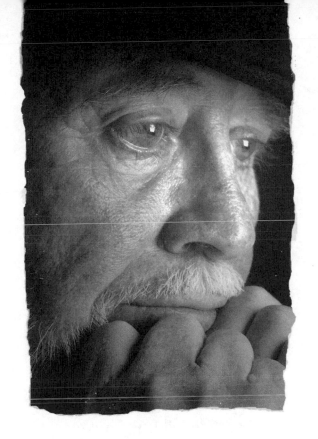

Chapter Four

Following:
The Magic of Palpation

If I dare to hear you, I will feel you like the sun and grow in your direction.

~ MARK NEPO, POET AND CANCER SURVIVOR

pal·pa·tion/pal-pey-shun/

A method of feeling with the hands during a physical examination; the act of examining something closely.

Palpation is one of the first things clinicians in health care learn. Because of the seductiveness and easy availability of technological means for diagnosing and monitoring our patients and the incredible pace of many health care institutions, there is a risk that this most fundamental skill will become one of the least exercised.

Most of us learned hands-on examination early in our education, and if we were lucky, we studied under or near someone who was very good at it. We found a new definition of thrill, and it was a thrill indeed to discover a murmur with just a stethoscope or to palpate a vein and know that you could access it for a blood draw or IV stick. We were invited to unravel the secret codes of pulses, and we saw how fluids inside reveal themselves on the outside.

Little did we realize, however, that this sharpening of our powers of observation would soon be used in a kind of palpation of our whole world. We started noticing facial expressions with the same care that we had learned to notice changes in skin color around a wound. Voice tones became as sharply differentiated and as meaningful to us as heart tones. We began to understand things around us sooner than others did because we were constantly collecting data without even thinking about it wherever we went. We were palpating the whole world around us.

We began to assess, even as we approached the patient's room, any unusual activity therein (the patient and his spouse are quietly arguing; the patient's breathing isn't right; something's funny on the monitor we haven't even looked at yet). Soon we were doing the same thing at home—quite unconsciously—or even as we walked from the car up the front walk: looking, hearing, smelling, noticing, considering, assessing.

In an article for athletic training educators, Eberman (2010) describes the process of learning palpation and practicing it until it becomes second nature:

> Learning palpation is like learning to read. At first, each word requires the identification of each letter, its phonetic value, and the linkages between each letter. As a person's ability to read increases, assessment of each word comes with more ease, patterns of words present themselves, and the significance of the sentence as a whole is appreciated....Once students have obtained these skills, they must develop the ability to organize their findings and relate them back to the patient's symptoms. Once a student is able to maneuver this process with ease, the act of palpation becomes intuitive. (p. 171)

Palpation is the primary component of the therapeutic practice of following. When we follow, we use already-acquired skills to attend to the rhythm and flow of the patient's words as much as to their content. We let each of the assessments we do every day build upon itself, one piece of revealed data suggesting what our next step or question should be. We allow ourselves to be guided by the revelation of the patient's verbal and nonverbal responses and the patient's teachings, just as we are guided by the revelations of the patient's body.

When we follow, we use already-acquired skills to attend to the rhythm and flow of the patient's words as much as to their content.

An elderly Irish nurse told us the story of her acquisition of this capacity. It was her first tutor in nursing school who reminded her to "use her eyes." He even declared that she couldn't legitimately call herself a nurse until she had learned how to do so. As it turned out, for Eleanor this would be just an extension of skills she learned on the farm. Michael turned her story into a meditation for the *See Me as a Person* CD (Trout, 2011).

"Use Your Eyes," He Said

He was our tutor,
and he told us that we could call ourselves "nurses"
only when we learned how to walk onto the unit
and learn—just by looking—the state of things:
what was different,
whose suffering had taken a turn,
who needed a kind word
or a bit of cheering up,
and who was becoming agitated
and would soon use up lots of our time
unless some small, preventive action were taken
right now.

It became my watchword.
"Use my eyes."
It's saved me a great deal of time all these years
and has defined me as the particular kind of caregiver
I am.

Perhaps I had a leg up on the other students
right out of the chute,
about this thing—
this sort of palpation of the unit
and palpation of the patient
without necessarily using my hands.

On the farm in Ireland
(just outside Killarney)
I worked beside my father.
(It was just the two of us,

as my mum had died when I was three.)
He didn't say a great deal,
but I quickly learned how to pay attention.
It was important to know how the cattle were doing
on a particular morning
before milking began.

(It might not go well, if I didn't.)
If the sow was cranky,
it might be best to catch on to the fact
before entering the pen
(unless I wanted to be chased around a bit).

It all came naturally to me.
I didn't have to work hard at it, I suppose,
and no one had to explain the importance of it.

Our life on that farm
depended on palpation,
on catching the rhythm of things.

Of course, I had always been a curious kid.
Everything interested me,
so paying attention hardly seemed a burden.
I felt joy in discovery.

And I never wasted much energy on judging folks.
Irascible and tough-minded as I am,
it just never made much sense to me
to look down on people who were already vulnerable.
The son of the folks on the neighboring farm
was seriously mentally ill,
but so what?
I watched him, because I was interested in him
not because he was a curiosity.
One time,

when I was sick,
he sent me a white rose.

Sometimes,
patients from the mental institution
in Killarney
would work on the farms near our village.
I was struck by these men,
whose grey faces
resembled their grey uniforms.
I was sad for them.
I thought they must not get enough fresh air
or something.
But it never occurred to me to think of them
as fundamentally different from me.

And so,
when faced with an angry patient
it wasn't hard for me to be more curious than fearful.
It wouldn't occur to me to tell an angry family member to
sit down
and stop fussing at me.
I'd want to know what it was
that had her upset.
So I would offer a cup of tea,
and we would sit for a minute,
often without saying too much.
And then she might tell me.
And the whole thing
would take less time than it would have
had I ignored the signs,
or tussled with her about who's in charge
and got the whole unit upset.

You don't order an agitated cow to settle down

(no matter how much you want to get on with the
milking).
You stop
and wonder about her
and maybe fix the problem
(the way the light's coming in the barn window
and flickering off that hay hook, into her eyes),
or maybe just sit on the butter box
and sing her a song.

I learned to notice things
when I was but a little girl.
I guess that all my tutor really did that day
was give direction to my natural curiosity
and my sense that this body of mine
was fully equipped to see,
touch,
hear,
and learn all about every place
I ever entered.

And,
yes,
I do call myself a nurse.
I've earned the title.

It is indeed a marvelous gift we have: this capacity for
palpation of everything around us.

The therapeutic practice of following is merely the intentional application of this gift as we pay attention and create a
transactional flow of information between ourselves and our
patients. In the process, we begin to create a relationship or to
deepen an existing one.

- Following refers to the practice of listening to, respecting, and acting on what we learn from our patients about who they are and what they want and need.

- Following means that we pay attention not only to the patient's words but also to voice tone, body language, facial expression, and gaze (including eye contact or lack thereof).

- Following means that we adjust our next caregiving act to align with what we are continually learning from the patient.

When we're following, we hook into the last thing the patient said or otherwise conveyed, and our next question follows what we've just learned from the patient. Because our actions follow the patient's or the patient's family's expressed wishes, the patient and family feel seen and valued, often not just by those who are doing such a good job of following in the moment, but by everyone in the organization and by the organization itself. Care becomes more intentionally customized to the needs and desires of our patients, and outcomes improve.

Following means that we learn about the patient's perspectives, experiences, history, culture, belief systems, even superstitions, and we decide to be guided by them. This does not necessarily mean that we suspend our knowledge about what is best, and we certainly don't suspend the delivery of care. Instead we include in our definition of care a curiosity about how the patient is experiencing our care, and we become curious about what it will take

Following means that we learn about the patient's perspectives, experiences, history, culture, belief systems, even superstitions, and we decide to be guided by them.

to support her ability to exercise free choice in determining aspects of her care.

When we practice following, the patient experiences himself as being in the hands of people who are interested in learning how to provide care that is specific to him. If the patient says that he was up all night, unable to breathe because of the antibiotic gel our protocol says must be pushed into his nostrils each evening, we follow: we ask, and so we discover, in this patient's case, that he is claustrophobic. Then we allow this information to influence our care of him as we reevaluate the infection-control protocol for this patient: Is it better for him to breathe and to sleep or to have every last possibility of infection kept at bay by filling his nose with antibiotics?

We look for nonverbal cues—especially for those moments in which the patient seems to be contradicting himself with his words and/or expressions. When the patient says "I'm fine," but she turns to face the wall, we follow: "You tell me you're fine, but your expression looks so sad. Is there something else?"

Following means that our questions are asked in earnest, and the responses are taken in as if they really matter, because they do. We show that they matter when we not only adjust our care, but we adjust our questions. Instead of limiting ourselves to a computer-based or memorized protocol, we let our subsequent questions build on the answers we've received so far. Suddenly our inquiries become organic, thoughtful, and thorough, and they serve their intended purpose: the acquisition of accurate, reliable, relevant information necessary to the provision of first-rate health care.

Following is the Most Effective Path to Leadership

Political leaders know it: in order to lead effectively, they must follow. They may forget the principle, but they do so at

138

their peril. They can only lead when they have paused and listened long enough to learn what the people are saying. They don't have to do exactly what they're told to do; indeed, this would be a path to chaos as there are so many voices speaking to them, but those who are successful know how to listen for and discern the core messages. If they choose to turn a deaf ear, they are soon turned out.

Parents also know that following is a big part of what makes them effective with their children. They get the most cooperation, the most buy-in for the day's plan, the most adherence to rules of the house, when they listen first. If Eric thinks the chore-sharing arrangements are unfair and tries to say so, his parents have a choice: ignore him ("Of course it's fair; what are you talking about?!"), which nearly assures he will do everything in his power to make chore day miserable for everyone; or they can hear him and let him know that they have heard him ("It sounds like you think Helen and Jenny hardly have to do anything,") which may open the door to compromise, negotiation, and actual agreement.

In both examples, despite the act of intentionally becoming a follower, the leader (the politician or the parent) never gives up the leadership role. The leader actually makes the role of leader work by following the people she plans to lead.

Certainly the politician can lead by saying, "I know best! I'm going to do what I like!" But she actually gives up her power with such a statement, not only because she looks like a tantrumming child (not much of a leader), but also because folks will, over time, learn to ignore her. The same goes for the parent, who most assuredly does not stop being a parent when he chooses to voluntarily offer his ear to his children in order to give them the sense that they have been involved in the formulation of the chore plan. He could say, of course, "I'm the parent, and I decide who does what." Many parents, fearful of handing over their power to their own children, say exactly this, but they actually disqualify themselves from being effective leaders by refusing to follow. They will be undermined; the only questions are when and how.

So when Ralphie runs into the kitchen whining, "Martha took my toy! She always does that!"—we parents have choices. We can set following aside and absent-mindedly respond, "Stop whining, Ralphie!" Or we can pay a little more attention—and still fail to follow—when we say, "I'm sure she didn't mean to take your toy, and I know she doesn't *always* do that. Anyway, you take her toys, too."

Both responses, since they miss the mark in acknowledging, showing empathy, or even catching on to what's happening from the child's perspective, will fail to address the problem and will make it nearly 100% certain that this particular problem will keep coming up.

Following Ralphie takes less energy than we think, and it actually conserves it over time because the problem begins to diminish. The following response doesn't have to be complicated, certainly doesn't have to be clinical, and doesn't require us to give up a thing. We just look at Ralphie, and let him know we heard him. When he tells us that Martha took his toy again, we say, simply: "She did?!"

"Yeah," says Ralphie. "I hate it when she does that!"

"You do?! Boy, you must be pretty mad." Ralphie nods, breathing a little easier.

Our following just shifted Ralphie's experience even though we have not even promised to help him. We just followed, and in our following we established exactly the sort of healing connection Ralphie wanted. But notice what else happened: we stayed in charge. We didn't take sides; we provided nothing more than a sturdy presence and a willingness to listen to what was distressing Ralphie, and with that small effort in following he is no longer obsessed with convincing us that Martha is a terrible sister. We already showed that we followed that idea; we "got it." He is free to move on to other things, as are we. We have led by following. It doesn't even matter that nothing got resolved. Mostly, Ralphie wanted to know that we heard him.

The funny thing is that we as health care professionals already know all about following. It's part of our technical expertise to do it every day. We never push ahead with our treatment agenda in the face of emerging evidence that something else needs our attention or that our treatment is exacerbating the situation. We make adjustments in our provision of technical care constantly, dynamically, in transaction with what we see, with what the patient's body teaches us. It never occurs to us to take personally what the body of our patient spits back at us by way of feedback regarding what we're doing.

When we can't stop the bleeding we don't hesitate for a moment to take responsibility for noticing the fact and taking immediate action to adjust to the information flowing out of the person's body. We don't ignore it; we don't get mad about it; and when we tell others about it in report, we do so with a mixture of clinical objectivity, deep involvement in solving the problem, and curiosity about its having happened. We find it interesting that things changed midstream and that we had to adjust.

We already knew there was nothing formulaic about the instrumental aspects of providing care. So why would we resist being similarly flexible, responsive, dynamic, curious, and robust in the relational aspects of our practice? Why would we be surprised, annoyed, defensive, or put-upon when the patient (or family member) tells us that we have been wrong, which requires an adjustment in our treatment? Why would our scientific curiosity and clinical dynamism not be aroused when manifestations of the illness include the patient being demanding, uncooperative, morose, thoughtless, or self-centered? Why would we not assume—just as we regularly do when we watch the patient's body for cues—that the patient's mind, soul, and voice have much to teach us about how he is doing and whether or not the specific care we're providing is hitting the mark?

When the bed-ridden patient begins to develop skin break-down we don't waste a moment with defensiveness (even though the new symptom is an effect of the treatment we are providing), with disgust (even though it's not too pretty), or with letting the patient know that this new demand of her body is a problem for us. We take in the new data and we act as only we know to act: with precision that is marked by responsiveness to what the patient has just taught us via her skin.

We respond to the situation. It's one of the things we do best. In order to respond, we have become world-class observers, voracious collectors of new information, changing speeds, changing approaches, all in a continuous transaction with the patient's symptoms. This is the formula for following that has become second nature for us in the instrumental aspects of care: watch, see, notice, wonder, record, and then act in accordance with what is in front of us.

It's a miracle of transaction. It's what is required of us in the instrumental aspects of our work, and it has been so since health care began. It's just that when we're following what the patient's body is telling us, that information is far less likely to make us weary or defensive than some of the information we're called to follow in the relational aspects of our work.

The next story is a case presentation offered by a health care clinician in one of our workshops. The comments that follow the initial case presentation represent the workshop participants' thoughts and our elaboration of them.

It's Never the Gravy

Everyone had just about had it with the patient in 407. Actually, it was not so much the patient as it was her sister who was always there and always complaining. But it had begun to affect everyone's attitude toward the patient herself. Sluggishness in response to the call light had become the norm because most of the time it wasn't even the patient using the call light; it was her demanding, impossible-to-satisfy sister.

The nurse enters. "Yes, Mrs. Jones?" she inquires, halfheartedly addressing the patient, but realizing the likelihood that it was her sister, Mrs. Hoffman, who had pushed the call light.

Just as the nurse suspected, Mrs. Jones had nothing to say—or at least she didn't get a chance to say it as her sister took over the interaction. "What kind of a place are you people running here? I've pressed this stupid call light six times in the last 15 minutes, and no one has even noticed! What does a patient have to do to get some action around here?"

"What is it we can help with?" the nurse inquires—not to the patient now, but to her sister—her body language signaling impatience if not exasperation.

"I've told every nurse I can find that my sister does not like gravy on her potatoes. Besides, it isn't good for her. Now they deliver dinner, once again, with—you guessed it—no sign whatsoever that anyone is listening to me. I'm trying to look after her. I'm the only one. It seems like I have to fight you for help in caring for her."

"I'm sorry dietary didn't get the message. They're very busy. Every dinner can't be custom-ordered, and it isn't nursing's job to examine the trays before they're delivered. Is there anything else I can do for you?" The nurse's words and affect are flat, so as to not encourage any further interaction; she is awaiting the moment when she can get out of there. She checks the IV drip, absent-mindedly tucks the patient's sheets around her, avoids eye contact with the sister, and departs.

Not exactly a satisfying encounter for the patient, the patient's sister, or the nurse.

The proof will be in the pudding, of course. If the patient felt comforted by the nurse's responses and the sister felt heard—in other words, if both of them experienced the nurse as following them—then things will get better. The sister's attitude will soften, her confidence in the hospital will rise, the patient will feel relaxed and able to focus her attention on healing, and the call light will get a chance to cool before it is pressed again.

Of course, none of that happened. No one felt followed, because, in fact, they were not followed. The nurse provided an answer to the sister's complaint, but her answer provided no comfort for Mrs. Jones. The patient remained agitated, and while her sister seemed to be the antagonist, the ultimate responsibility for putting the patient in a position to get better lies with the people responsible for her care. It lies with the understandably worn-down nurse who is caring for her on this particular shift.

The truth is that things will not get better after the intervention described above. Indeed, experience teaches us that this unheard, unacknowledged sister is now officially at war. This hospital is now her enemy, and the nursing staff are in the crosshairs. She cannot trust that her sister will receive good care. She will accelerate her demands, staff members will be further drained, and the energy of the unit will suffer. Mrs. Hoffman's sister—the actual patient—is going to be affected by the toxic interactions between her sister and just about everybody else; the optimal conditions for her healing will be unavailable to her.

But what would happen for the patient, the sister, and even the unit if the nurse practiced following?

"Yes, Mrs. Jones?" This time, the nurse looks as though she means these words as a sincere question. This time she seems interested in what Mrs. Jones (or anyone else who's concerned about her care) has to say. Her body says so. Her face says so. Her voice says so. Even her physical placement in the room— the proximity she establishes to the patient and her sister—says so.

While following means giving careful attention to the body language, voice tone, and affect of the patient, it also means paying attention to your own body language, facial expressions, voice tone, touch, words, and empathetic sounds. With her mostly silent, sincere attentiveness she conveys, in effect: "I am here to look after you. Right now, 'you' includes your family member. Tell me what I need to know in order to give you the very best care possible."

Paradoxically, this new posture also establishes her as the leader; she has suddenly taken back the conversation by agreeing to be led by it. She has regained her authority, and even her emotional distance from the problem, by immersing herself in it.

Still determined to drive the conversation but taken aback, the sister softens a bit. After all, she doesn't have to fight to get her audience anymore. The audience appeared and seemed quite interested in her. The sister's words begin with stridency (after all, she was not prepared for someone who was sincerely curious about her thoughts): "What kind of a place are you people running here? I've pressed this stupid call light six times in the last 15 minutes, and no one has even noticed! What does a patient have to do to get some action?"

"Oh, Mrs. Hoffman. That's not okay. If you were pressing the call light so many times, you must have been very worried about your sister."

"Uh, yes. That's right. So, what's the problem around . . . " Her voice trails off as if she momentarily forgot what she was so upset about. She is taken off guard by nothing more than the nurse's simple curiosity. Someone is paying attention to her concerns without defensiveness.

"So, tell me how I can help."

"It's the gravy. I told them no gravy, but you keep giving her gravy. I don't think it's good for her . . . and anyway, she doesn't really like . . . " The steam seems to have gone out of her engines.

"I can see that you're really watching out for your sister's health, and you must think sometimes that we're not."

"Well, I'm sure you try, but . . . you just don't realize how much I worry . . . "

"I think I'm beginning to understand that you have a big responsibility. Would you go for a walk with me? We'll go tell dietary together. Maybe that will help."

The nurse knew, of course, that the issue was not the gravy. (Most clinicians know that the issue is never the gravy.)

It doesn't matter, though. Really, this master of attunement, this leader of a nurse, this one who came to give the most important thing she has today—her attention—has taken charge. She asks the sister to accompany her out of the room for a minute so she can hear this concerned family member better.

Not quite making it to dietary, they stop by a window overlooking the park. They are both quiet for a moment, staring at the sky together. Mrs. Hoffman speaks first.

"When our mom died, her last words to me were to look after my sister and brother. I wasn't surprised; since I was the oldest, I always had looked after them. When we were little Mom worked two jobs to be able to support us, which meant I was the designated babysitter much of the time. Once Julie walked off while I wasn't paying enough attention. It scared me to death. When mom came home and found out, she told me that if anything ever happened to Julie, she would never forgive me."

"Ohhh," the nurse breathes, looking directly into Mrs. Hoffman's eyes, "That's a great deal of responsibility. I can see that you take your promise to your mother very seriously."

As they walk on, no longer intent on making it to dietary, Mrs. Hoffman murmurs, "I could just scrape the gravy off." Quietly, they turn around and head back to the room. At the door, Mrs. Hoffman touches the nurse's arm and says simply, "Thank you."

You can guess the outcome of this brief moment of following. Over the next several days, all of the staff benefit with savings in time and energy from this modest investment in following by one attuned, present nurse. The number of demands rumbling out of 407 plummets. Neither Mrs. Jones nor her suddenly calmed, understood, and seen sister, ever treat the call light like their own private maid service again. The unit feels different. The attitudes of the clinical staff change in response to the new feeling in room 407. Report is different regarding this patient. Mrs. Hoffman becomes a true collaborator in her sister's care, actually providing invaluable assistance to the nursing staff.

The actions of the nurse in the second scenario (much like the earlier actions of the parent who follows Ralphie) illustrate that following is leading. Leadership at its core is about our ability to help the other become more able to cope, to succeed, and to be whole. The nurse in the second scenario promised nothing, and in fact, she delivered nothing except for the one thing Mrs. Hoffman wanted: she was truly present with her; she listened. Her aim was simply to be present with the person in front of her and to respond authentically to what she observed. Her intention was to follow, and following, all by itself, was enough.

Following is Conscious Listening

Therapeutic listening requires levels of awareness and presence that are not easy to achieve. French philosopher Simone Weil (1951/2009) wrote, "The capacity to give one's attention to a sufferer is a rare and difficult thing; it is almost a miracle; it *is* a miracle. Nearly all those who think they have the capacity do not possess it" (p. 64).

Why is therapeutic listening so difficult? What prevents us from being fully present and listening? What are the implications if Weil is correct—that many of us think we possess this ability but we actually don't? What are the conditions that most help us to follow and truly listen to a person, taking in his words, his emotions, and his nonverbal cues? We can only begin to answer these questions for ourselves through honest self-reflection. We may also find clues to our own listening "blind spots" by asking close colleagues, friends, and members of our own families to tell us how they perceive our listening capacity and what may get in our way when we listen to them.

There are some classic obstacles to therapeutic listening listed below. A common thread through all of these obstacles is our well-documented drive for self-protection (Jourard, 1971; Rogers, 1951; Warner, 2001). If we feel threatened and defensive by the intensity of the situation, by the possibility of conflict, by feelings of helplessness or fear of not knowing, it becomes difficult for us to remain open, receptive, and curious— all prerequisites for true listening. What follows is a list of the

What are the conditions that most help us to follow and truly listen to a person, taking in his words, his emotions, and his nonverbal cues?

practices that clinicians may reflexively turn to instead of conscious listening, in the face of our own emotional discomfort or even the always-looming potential for it.

1) Fixing

As health care clinicians, fixing is our stock-in-trade. We listen with a "fixing ear," perhaps habitually listening for problems we can solve decisively. One obvious problem with our tendency to rush in and fix is that we shut down our access to the full range of important information. Also, if we were to quietly reflect on who we were actually making feel better by fixing, it may be apparent that it was our own discomfort with expressions of suffering (fear, anger, ambiguity, tears) that moved us into a fixing mode.

2) Advising

A close relative to fixing, advising may prematurely shut down the ability or willingness of the other to express himself. We know we are advising when we hear ourselves saying "I think you should . . . " or "If I were you . . . " or "Why don't you . . . ." Like fixing, advising appears to benefit the patient, but it's worth reflecting on who it may be serving most.

3) Educating

Education is a necessary intervention in health care. It is fundamental to people learning what they need to know in order to manage their health conditions. Yet, like advising and fixing, it can become an obstacle to listening if it is commenced prematurely and interrupts the other's expression before she is ready. Education becomes an obstacle when it is seen as the solution before what will actually work for this particular person is thoroughly listened to, considered, and understood.

(Remember baby James' mom from Chapter 3, when the well-meaning physician launched right into changing the young mother's feeding style without fully listening to her?) If there is not a readiness to learn and education is forced, the intervention is not likely to be successful.

4) Story-telling

For some listeners it can be extremely challenging to refrain from telling their own story when listening to another. These listeners may believe that the sharing of their own story of a similar experience is an effective way to create a connection with the other person. Unfortunately, it's far more likely to interrupt the focus on the other and redirect attention away from the person back to the clinician. Admittedly, there may be some rare instances in which sharing a small part of your story is appropriate and helpful. (It may take this form: "My mother had a similar diagnosis three years ago. This must be very difficult for you, too." Then become quiet; because your intention is to open the other up, not to share your story.) If your intention is to use a brief story that stirs the person to open more, you are likely on a therapeutic track. If your intention is to let him know about you, to convince him you understand him, or to convey your knowledge, you are likely departing from a therapeutic focus.

5) Distancing and shutting down

Some people cope with others' expressions of intense emotions and behaviors such as anger and criticism by shutting down and becoming unable to be emotionally receptive. One patient described this behavior this way: "The nurse's eyes suddenly became flat and empty . . . she was there in body, but it was like my words were falling into empty space. She was simply holding on until I stopped talking. She then muttered something I could not hear and left the room." Family therapist Michael Nichols (1995) calls this "listening with a clenched mind" (p.154).

6) Explaining or correcting

Our tendency to stop listening and explain what happened or to correct another's perceptions is closely linked to our need to be seen as competent, capable, and perhaps even in charge. When we do so, however, we shut down the other. As with some of the other obstacles, we may gain short-term control of the situation, but the price is high as we leave the person feeling unseen, unheard, and misunderstood.

7) Excessive responding

Similar to telling our own stories, excessive interrupting and questioning can masquerade as interest and curiosity. Excessive expressions of support such as *wow, oh my goodness, that's awful, I know what you mean*, etc., can at first make it appear that the listener is tuned in to the other's feelings. However, when it is overdone, interfering with the speaker's ability to express and stay on track, it is disruptive and the speaker does not feel seen or heard. Excessive responding, like the other obstacles, shifts the focus from the speaker to the listener.

Self-Assessment: Conscious Listening

Conscious listening is fundamental to following. Like all of the therapeutic practices and skills, it requires that we cultivate our capacity to be present and aware and that we encounter each person with new eyes and ears.

It helps if we remember that an empathetic, therapeutic response is most frequently a quiet or even silent one. We encourage people to express themselves through our nonverbal invitations and encouragement and through our clear interest, respect, and regard. To mature in our development as conscious listeners we need to become aware of and understand our own blind spots. The following self-assessment was adapted from the writing of Michael Nichols in his book, *The Lost Art of Listening* (1995, pp. 61-74). It is a useful tool for evaluating your strengths and identifying areas for focus and development.

1.	I suspend my own agenda and seek to understand the other person.	Yes No Sometimes
2.	I do not rush to fix or give advice.	Yes No Sometimes
3.	I refrain from telling my own experience, recognizing that it disrupts my ability to follow the speaker and shifts the focus to me.	Yes No Sometimes
4.	I give the other person sufficient time to say what's on his or her mind, and I follow and acknowledge his or her experience.	Yes No Sometimes
5.	I refrain from being an excessive responder, interrupting to express my reaction or to express sympathy or to interrogate.	Yes No Sometimes
6.	I remember that an empathetic response is often restrained and largely silent, encouraging the speaker to go deeper.	Yes No Sometimes
7.	When others are worried or upset, I know that telling them not to feel the way they do or reassuring them that they need not worry is not helpful and may shut them down. I acknowledge their feelings and make room for them to talk as they choose.	Yes No Sometimes
8.	I am aware of my own emotional triggers and scan for biases and/or judgments that may interfere with my ability to be an open and responsive listener.	Yes No Sometimes

9. I demonstrate a willingness to listen without defending, criticizing, or correcting.	Yes No Sometimes
10. I inquire and clarify to make sure I understand the meaning of the other.	Yes No Sometimes

Conscious Listening May Include the Artful Use of Empathetic Sounds

Paralinguistics is the study of vocal communication that is separate from actual language. It includes examination of such things as voice tone, inflection, pitch, speed, intensity, and even the use of silence. If you think about the powerful effect a tone of voice or silence can have on the meaning of an interaction, it becomes apparent that this area of communication is extremely important to the therapeutic process. Based on a person's tone of voice or use of silence, we may feel safe, seen, accepted, and respected. In contrast, when presented with the very same words or silences conveyed in a different tone of voice we may feel threatened, unsafe, marginalized, and disrespected. The effect of these paralinguistic elements will depend almost entirely on how closely they follow what is being offered by the other person.

As we practice following, we pay attention to the nonverbal cues of the people we care for. We listen for words and we listen for meaning through both the verbal and nonverbal (yet audible) vocal cues that others offer to us, and we need to be equally aware of our own verbal and nonverbal audible vocal cues. Consider for a moment the almost infinite things we could mean by the simple utterance, "hmmmm . . . ."

In our work with health care clinicians, they often voice concern about what to do or what to say in the face of intense emotional circumstances. Remembering that presence is, in and of itself, a therapeutic intervention, we can then remember that it's less about what we say and more about how present we are, the way in which we are listening, the degree to which we are following, and the myriad ways in which we are conveying that the person has our undivided attention. Just allowing what the person has said to register on your face in a way that is clearly empathetic can be an effective therapeutic expression of following.

It is difficult to convey this idea about nonverbal, yet audible vocal expressions of empathy, and yet we know it when we experience it. We call it the art of the empathetic sound. It is an empathetic sigh, a quiet, "oh . . . ," a hum that means "I am so sorry," but it is vocalized without words.

One patient receiving mental health services to help her recover from a tragic loss in her life described the power of two words expressed by her therapist with an empathetic sigh. She said the words were much less like an actual verbal phrase and more like an out-breath of compassion and validation. He would say simply, "Of course" as in, "Of course you feel the way you do . . . ," which conveyed to her that there was validity in what she was feeling in response to her circumstances. When he sighed those two words she felt soothed, validated, and no longer alone in her struggles. She said that those two words—the empathetic and validating sound of them—made her feel connected, courageous, and perhaps most importantly, normal.

Laurence Savett, a physician and author of *The Human Side of Medicine: Learning What It's Like to be a Patient and What It's Like to be a Physician* (2002), describes the importance of conveying empathy through the use of empathetic sounds. He says that when he was a young and less experienced physician his inclination was to provide remedy (the quick fix) without first acknowledging the patient's feelings, struggles, and reactions to their circumstances. He heard a story from a rabbi that helped him remember the importance of empathy first, and this insight has guided his practice ever since.

> *Two boys, the son of a rabbi and his best friend, decide to play a game. "You be the rabbi," says the son of the rabbi, "and I'll be his congregant." "Rabbi," the boy-congregant says, "I'm having trouble in my marriage, trouble with my boss, and trouble with my daughter." Replies the boy-rabbi, "You should pay more attention to your wife, confront your boss, and make peace with your daughter." To which the rabbi's son replies, "No, no, no, you didn't do it right. You didn't first say, 'Oy!'" (p. 167)*

Savett clarifies that the first word out of his mouth after listening to patients' stories is not necessarily, "oy!" but it has been an "oy equivalent."

Pay attention to your expression of empathetic sounds. The old adage that less is more works when it comes to walking through high-intensity experiences with patients and their loved ones. Quiet presence, regard for the other, and conveying your empathy through nonverbal and empathetic sounds will serve you and the one you are caring for well.

Following is Responsive Touch

One example in which a caregiving behavior requires exquisite following is the use of touch. Touch is powerful nonverbal communication. If touch is used as a result of following and occurs in the context of careful attention to the requirements of following, it can be nurturing, responsive, uplifting, comforting, reassuring, and healing. When touch is used outside the context of following it can become intrusive, invasive, disconcerting, distracting, or even assaultive.

We know that touch is essential for our survival and that it is an important aspect of healing and care. Just as empathetic sounds convey meaning and empathy that words may not, an appropriate touch can ease pain and facilitate connection. Seasoned clinicians are often masters at following cues and knowing when to touch, how much to touch, and whether to touch at all. Yet most acknowledge that they received little formal education on the topic of touching and tending to the human body. Most clinicians are taught about touching the body from the perspective of objectivity and routine procedures. The emphasis is on getting the job done and protecting all involved from embarrassment by learning appropriate ways to drape, protecting the patient's privacy by closing curtains, adopting a matter-of-fact attitude, and remaining affectively neutral.

Jocalyn Lawler, an Australian nurse sociologist, conducted a study specific to the "intimacy of nursing practice and the human body" (1991, p. 3). She refers to this arena of practice as the "problem of the body," and she explores the ways, the meaning, and the impact for the patient and the caregiver of having "privileged access to other people's bodies" (p. 4). In her book, *Behind the Screens* (1991), she proposes that the reason little is formally taught and very little has been researched about the privilege of accessing people's bodies is that the topic of touching the body is taboo—something we just don't want to talk much about. She says that touching and tending to a person's body can be experienced as "embarrassing, threatening, frightening, and unfamiliar for the patients—but also for the clinicians themselves, especially those new to the clinical role" (p. 5). The purpose of her work is to make this fundamental human aspect of caregiving visible and knowledge-based.

Her research questions in and of themselves are both compelling and provocative in their ability to stimulate a greater consciousness and understanding about this domain of care. With greater consciousness comes a greater likelihood that we will follow and touch patients with sensitivity. Thus, we included this area of touch explicitly and have adapted some of Lawler's research questions for your reflection below (1991, p. 7):

- What methods have you learned to facilitate your work of caring for the human body when your care is invasive of the body and therefore gives rise to potential and actual embarrassment?

- How do you negotiate the social territory of doing for patients what they would normally do for themselves in private?

- How do you facilitate patients' emotional safety when you must touch parts of their body that could result in embarrassment or heightened feelings of vulnerability?

- What guides the way you touch and care for a dying patient and the body after death?

- How do you help people cope with a dysfunctional, disfigured, deformed, or damaged body?

- What does it take for you to care for others when the tasks to be performed are potentially or actually nauseating or truly awful?

- How do you recognize embarrassment (your own or the patient's) and cope with it?

Necessary Touch versus Comforting, Supporting Touch

It could be said that there are two types of touch when caring for a person: 1) necessary touch, which is fairly simple to understand, and 2) comforting and supporting touch, which is infinitely nuanced in its complexity.

Necessary Touch

When the patient must be touched during a procedure, we prepare the person to be touched and ask permission. The touch is necessary, so the permission is sought and the person is invited to participate in how that touch will be handled. Because it's a human-to-human interaction, it too will be nuanced, but this is a relatively straightforward piece of the touch dynamic.

Because necessary touch is part of care, it can become habitual and formulaic; we can become unconscious about it. However, even this relatively straightforward use of touch requires awareness and must not be routinized. In a clinical setting no touch is routine for patients.

If we are not mindful, touch that we may consider routine can result in an extremely negative response from the patient, as in the following example. A young chemotherapy patient was being seen in the clinic by her primary physician. She had been suffering for several days from a painful rash along one side of her body. As she was being admitted, the nursing assistant took the young woman by the arm as she stepped on the scale to be weighed. The young girl screamed out in pain and the nursing assistant, embarrassed and caught off-guard, responded, "I didn't hurt you! I was just trying to help you up on onto the scale." The young woman began to cry. She was diagnosed later in this same visit with an advanced case of shingles, a side effect of her chemotherapy, and she was started on antiviral treatment.

There is no telling why the nursing assistant's response was triggered by the young woman's cry of pain at her truly gentle touch. It's human nature to want people to respond in predictable, reasonable ways, and in this case the patient's response startled the nursing assistant and threw her off balance. When our gentle touch provokes an unexpected reaction, however, it's helpful if we begin wondering and following rather than reacting to the "unreasonableness" of the patient's response. Preferably the nursing assistant would have initiated the contact by saying, "May I help you onto the scale?" before touching the patient, but after the incident, having missed her first opportunity for following, she could still have offered following in response to the girl's startling reaction to her touch. "I'm so sorry. I didn't mean to hurt you. Tell me what's going on."

Not surprisingly, there is much to be learned about touch by looking at the healing modality of massage therapy. In massage therapy it's understood that the patient is vulnerable—sometimes in pain, typically naked, and facing down with eyes closed—and that no touch should ever be unexpected. A friend told us of an experience in massage therapy training in which she and her fellow students agreed to be blindfolded and then to interact with each other in a small, closed room. In this exercise they discovered how jarring it is to be touched unexpectedly, even as able-bodied, fully clothed persons who had agreed to the interaction. As jarring as it was for them, it's exponentially more jarring for our patients who, in many instances, are already on high alert physically and emotionally because of the pain they're in or the procedures that have been done to them and the ongoing invasions of their bodies throughout the course of their care.

We preserve our patients' dignity when, rather than imposing our touch on them, we offer it:

- "I'm going to ask you to turn onto your side, and I'll hold your blanket to cover you." Wait for the patient's response, and then follow it.

- "I'm going to need to start an IV; may I hold your arm now?" Wait for the patient's response, and then follow it.

- "May I help you onto the scale?" Wait for the patient's response, and then follow it.

When touch is respectful rather than presumptive, it enhances care. When it's presumptive, it may be a way to control the patient or distance ourselves from his pain. When touch is presumptive, the therapeutic relationship is compromised and trust can be shaken.

Comforting and Supporting Touch

When there is no instrumental reason to touch the patient, knowing when to use touch to comfort another or give support requires a mix of intuition and observation; it requires following.

In much the same way that paralinguistic utterances can have multiple meanings, touch is sometimes understood in exactly the way it's intended, but it also has the potential to be misunderstood completely. Also like paralinguistic utterances, the manner of the caregiver has a profound effect on how her touch is perceived by the patient. If the clinician is placing a hand on the arm of the patient during a procedure that the patient seems to be distressed about, the patient may take that to mean, "It's okay; I'm here," but the patient may also perceive the hand on her arm to mean, "Stop moving so much," or "Calm down." This is why it's vitally important to scan yourself for any agenda before you reach your hand out toward another to administer touch.

It's vitally important to scan yourself for any agenda before you reach your hand out toward another to administer touch.

Are you willing to be with the other in his or her pain?

A daughter watches as her aging mother, seeming daily to shrink smaller and smaller in the hospital bed, is seized with sudden acute chest pains. The daughter is asked to leave the room while clinicians tend to the emergency. She feels kicked out—ostracized and abandoned. Does she want to be touched? Even she wouldn't know the answer to that question if it were asked with words, but when a social worker who observed her abrupt dismissal from the room as her mother seized in pain walks over to the daughter, puts his hand on the daughter's shoulder, and says gently, "This is really difficult," the daughter, relieved to discover that she is no longer isolated in her own suffering, leans into the social worker, allowing him to take just a little bit of the overwhelming weight she's been carrying since the beginning of her mother's illness and undeniable decline.

This social worker could not have known conclusively that the daughter would welcome his touch, but he had done some following, so he was able to perceive that, based on his own intuition and what he observed, touch would be welcome. He noticed that the daughter herself touched her mother as she spoke to her. The social worker also noted as he approached the daughter that she looked up responsively and appeared through her body language and cues to be open to and in fact needful of physical comforting, and therefore, would be responsive to his shoulder touch.

The risk of using therapeutic touch in a purely relational way is that it can most certainly be rejected, but the reward is that it can heal things we didn't even realize needed healing. There's always the chance that he might have misread the daughter, but this compassionate social worker would then have removed his hand and just stayed present.

As is true with all of our human interactions, there is not a precise formula for touching. However, we have outlined four clinical considerations regarding touch that may be useful as general guidelines:

1. Remember that while touch is necessary for administering care, it is never experienced as routine

by the person receiving care. Touch is a privileged access to the body.

2. Our backgrounds and experiences determine how we will respond to touch. We learn what works for each person by wondering and following.

3. Surprise touch can be jarring. Prepare the patient for touch and ask permission.

4. Mindful touch, based on following, facilitates healing and recovery.

It takes confidence and even courage to touch therapeutically. There's no telling whether the nursing assistant who touched the arm of the young woman with shingles will become more mindful as she touches patients; or if she will abandon touch almost completely, using it only when it's unavoidable; or if she might learn nothing, framing the whole incident as an overdramatic response from the patient. When your touch is rejected, it's not personal. The patient with shingles was giving the nurse information with her outcry. As startling as it was, it was information, not condemnation.

In our own experience we have also found that, for the majority of patients, feeling as though others are avoiding touching them is just as difficult as receiving unexpected touch. In a world where so many of our interactions with patients are "gloved," people can begin to feel like pariahs even as they recognize and appreciate the importance of preventing cross-contamination and infections. When they don't receive the mindful touch they need—and especially when measures are visibly taken to avoid touching them—people may feel untouchable and isolated, and healing may be compromised. A facilitator of the workshop *Re-Igniting the Spirit of Caring* told us this story about a former patient who came to share her care experience with the health care professionals participating in the workshop.

Protective Isolation

A middle-aged female patient came to one of our workshops to participate in the patient caring panel, and before she began her story, she looked across the room and pointed to a nurse in the rear corner table and said, "You probably don't remember me, but I'll never forget you. It was 12 or 13 years ago when you took care of me when I was a patient on your floor."

The nurse appeared confused and a little embarrassed, but admitted she didn't recognize this patient.

The patient continued, "I was in protective isolation, and isolation is the right word. I felt so isolated, depressed, and lonely, like I had leprosy or something. Everyone who came into my room wore gowns, gloves, and masks, and I wasn't sure who was who some of the time.

But I'll never forget you. You took off a glove and touched me and held my hand, and when I felt the warmth of your touch and your skin touching mine, something changed inside of me, and I felt hope for the first time. That's why I'll never forget you and how your caring made such a difference to me."

It was very hard to re-group and continue after the impact of that moment. I remember no one wanted to speak and break the honoring of the story and the intense emotional effect of that brief healing moment that lived so richly in the memory of this patient after more than twelve years had passed.

The following poem by Marge Piercy (2010) captures the profound truth that touch is a core human craving. From birth to death we are sustained, and in fact sometimes we are kept alive, by touch.

The tao of touch

What magic does touch create
that we crave it so. That babies
do not thrive without it. That
the nurse who cuts tough nails
and sands calluses on the elderly
tells me sometimes men weep
as she rubs lotion on their feet.

Yet the touch of a stranger
the bumping or predatory thrust
in the subway is like a slap.
We long for the familiar, the open
palm of love, its tender fingers.
It is our hands that tamed cats
into pets, not our food.

The widow looks in the mirror
thinking, no one will ever touch
me again, never. Not hold me.
Not caress the softness of my
breasts, my inner things, the swell
of my belly. Do I still live
if no one knows my body?

We touch each other so many
ways, in curiosity, in anger,
to command attention, to soothe,
to quiet, to rouse, to cure.
Touch is our first language
and often, our last as the breath
ebbs and a hand closes our eyes.

The Power of Following the Nonverbal Cue

This story, told to us by Maria Bellchambers (personal communication, June 14, 2011) is about how very subtle following can be.

"You Wouldn't Leave Me Alone"

I can still see his face. He was so sad.

He wasn't my patient, but whenever I walked past his door, I looked in, as any ICU nurse does. We're always in a state of alert.

Every time I walked past the room he was alone. He was all shut down and blank in the eyes, but his face was turned toward the door. This was unusual, because the tendency is that when patients shut down they turn their backs to the door. I don't know that it really registered fully with me at the time that this small detail was somehow an opening—a tiny invitation to make a connection. Certainly everything else about his scowling affect was resolutely uninviting.

Still, he was always facing the door.

One time as I walked by I caught his eyes. I pulled up a chair so that my face was level with his. I would talk with him—just pleasantries at first, "Hi, how are you, how is your day..." He would respond in Chinese, knowing that I wouldn't understand it. He wouldn't talk to anyone in our language even though he'd been educated here and spoke it fluently.

I'd never seen him with a visitor, but I'd heard that his parents had come at one point. They were reported to be very disappointed with him. He'd attempted suicide (and came very close to succeeding) because his grades hadn't been good enough to get him into the college his parents had wanted him to attend. Now, in his estimation, he'd failed his family not once but twice—first with his unacceptable grades and then with the further humiliation of a suicide attempt that was too close to successful to sweep under the rug.

I felt sad for him. He didn't have to choose to live this way. I believed there was hope for him.

It didn't matter that he never responded to me. I would just sit next to him and talk. "I know things didn't go your way," I'd say to him. Sometimes he was blank-faced, and sometimes he would glare at me. I told him, "I have seen patients come in devastated and walk out of here and go on to live very fruitful lives and have families, children who loved them." He responded but not a lot. I told him, "You can choose to be the author of your own life." Every now and then his eyes would catch my eyes and I had glimpses of looking into him.

Three years later I was at a restaurant in my town with a friend and a young man came up to me. He said, "You don't remember me, do you? You're a nurse, right?" "I am a nurse," I said, "but I don't remember you."

"You talked me out of committing suicide," he said. I thought about it—I'd never talked anyone out of committing suicide. I pictured someone on a ledge and myself talking him out of jumping.

Then I recognized his eyes.

"You tortured me," he teased gently. "You kept coming back. You kept coming into my room, and many times I was planning how I was going to kill myself. Every time I thought I had a plan, you sat down and started talking to me. You wouldn't leave me alone. You kept saying that I could be the author of my own life."

His life is good now. He has a girlfriend. He's in a community college. Back when he was in the ICU he had told his family to stop visiting, knowing that when they would come he would feel worse. I asked if his parents were in his life now. "It's okay now. I don't see them too much because I'm doing what I want to do."

It was incredibly humbling, that meeting in the restaurant.

The young man gave Maria very little tangible feedback, but she trusted her intuition that there was some tiny, almost imperceptible invitation in this young man's way of being with her. Had something in him given a signal to something in her?

Perhaps in some way the young man was giving Maria something to follow, and perhaps her receptivity to what he was giving her lives outside of what we think of as normal cognitive consciousness. As we deepen our experience with the practice of following, we're likely to learn that the need of one calling to another is sometimes profoundly silent.

In Michael's practice as a child and family therapist, he works with a particular kind of child who is especially difficult for foster or adoptive parents to reach. Such children, who often present superficially as confident and charming, are actually terrified and riddled with shame. They resist genuine human connection. Traditional talk therapies or play therapies are useless. These children are streetwise, smart, and they utterly confound their parents' management strategies at home.

The beleaguered, frustrated, emotionally-depleted parents drag these children in to therapy, but they can't make them talk about anything they don't want to talk about or anything that really matters to them. The road to meaningful conversation is closed, but even in those cases, connection is sometimes possible through the simple practice of following.

Connection is sometimes possible through the simple practice of following.

Connection by way of following requires complete suspension of any goal other than the goal of helping the child feel seen. The child may come in dragging his feet, walking 15 feet behind his parent, looking at the floor, and refusing eye contact. Michael will say something about what he's wearing, his hair, or merely state out loud what is obvious to all: he doesn't want to be here!

That's it: just following and more following. If we're very lucky, over time some small movement toward connection with an outside world perceived by the child as rejecting, disinterested, and hostile, can be made. Meanwhile, the parents (who are usually at the end of their rope by the time they come to Michael) are starting to notice: things sometimes happen when they give up the agenda, when they stop giving moral lessons, when they stop focusing on behavior and they just see the child, right where he is, just as he is.

Sometimes, after nothing whatsoever has happened clinically except that the therapist focuses on following, the sullen child squeaks out a thought: "You wish you never got me."

All clinicians know this experience or some version of it. There are times when direct questions don't get us anywhere. In those instances we just follow because that's the only thing we have that can move us toward any connection at all. All other doors to building a relationship are closed.

It's important to note, though, that following isn't a strategy. Following, in and of itself, as Maria's story so beautifully demonstrates, is a healing modality. We don't follow in order to get information or cooperation or gratitude or higher customer service scores. We follow to connect. Like the young man in Maria's story who was unresponsive to her for his entire time in the ICU, some people may never express that you're making any difference for them at all. Still, connection can make a bigger difference than we could possibly imagine, perhaps especially for those who give us every indication that connection is not what they want.

Language for Following

The language of following includes paying attention to and responding directly to both verbal and nonverbal cues. It means tailoring your communication to what people are saying with words as well as what they're saying with their bodies. It also includes being aware of your own body language and empathetic words and sounds. Some examples of the language of following are provided in the box below:

Verbal Following Language

When you _____, I noticed _____.

Tell me more about _____.

Tell me what is happening now ....

When you said _____, I wondered _____.

What was that like for you, for your family?

You seem (sad, excited, worried, etc.); is that true?

Is there more about _____ that you would like me to know?

Let's see if I have this right: you _____; is that accurate?

What is most important to you about _____?

Nonverbal Following Language

Body Posture:
- Open
- Attuned
- Leaning toward
- Appropriate proximity
- Appropriate eye contact
- Appropriate touch

Empathetic Sounds:
- Authentic vocalization ("oy equivalents")
- Soothing sounds
- Affirmative sounds ("of course ...")

Summary of Key Thoughts

- We are palpating the whole world around us. We notice facial expressions with the same care that we have learned to notice changes in skin color around a wound. Voice tones became as sharply differentiated—and as meaningful to us—as heart tones.

- Much like what we know as palpation, following refers to the practice of listening to, respecting, and acting on what we learn from our patients about who they are and what they want and need. Following is an ongoing practice.

- Following means that we adjust our next caregiving act to align with what we are noticing, allowing ourselves always to be guided by what the patient teaches us about who she is and what she wants and needs.

- Following is learning about the person's perspective and consciously allowing yourself to be guided by it.

- Following is listening.

- Following does not ask that you provide solutions—only that you connect with the person based on the information, both verbal and nonverbal, that he provides.

- While following means giving careful attention to the body language, voice tone, and affect of the patient, it also means paying attention to your own body language, voice tone, touch, words, and empathetic sounds.

- Following is leading. Despite the act of intentionally becoming a follower, the clinician never gives up the leadership role. The clinician actually makes the role of leader work by following the people he plans to lead.

- Leadership at its core is about our ability to help the other become more able to cope, to succeed, and to be whole.

- We as health care professionals do one sort of following all day every day, as following the cues of the body is actually a fundamental part of the technical aspect of care.

- One of the most important aspects of following is that we take in and remember information about our patients without losing our sense of wonder about them, without pigeonholing them based on the information they give us. We must allow our patients to be continually "new" as their situations change over time.

- By following the patient and family, we deepen our relationship with them as following requires us to be authentic in our interactions.

- Following is not a strategy; it is a healing modality.

Reflection

- Simone Weil said, "The capacity to give one's attention to a sufferer is a rare and difficult thing . . . Nearly all who think they have the capacity do not possess it." What do you think about this statement? What gives you the strength to give your attention to people who are suffering? What, if anything, hinders you?

- "Following, in and of itself, is a healing modality." Do you agree with this statement? Why or why not?

- Reflect on the ways you follow in your care of patients and their loved ones. Is there a way you can do more of it and/or do it more effectively?

- Reflect on Jocalyn Lawler's seven research questions on the privilege of touching the human body on page 157. They are provocative in nature, as the body is often considered a taboo subject even though many caregivers interact with the body constantly. Avoiding this topic limits our awareness and also inhibits our ability to learn from and teach each other. Determine which of these questions you want to explore personally and/or with a group and engage in conversation about them.

- Listen to "'Use Your Eyes,' He Said," (found on the *See Me as a Person* CD) with a group of colleagues and reflect together on what it means to you and your practice.

- Notice your own experience with touching and being touched. Notice cues from those in your care as you engage in both necessary touch and comforting touch.

- Beginning on page 149, there are seven classic obstacles to therapeutic listening. Identify one that you specifically want to work on in order to strengthen your ability to follow.

- What strengths have you identified in your listening assessment on page 152? Identify one or two listening habits that you will strengthen in your practice.

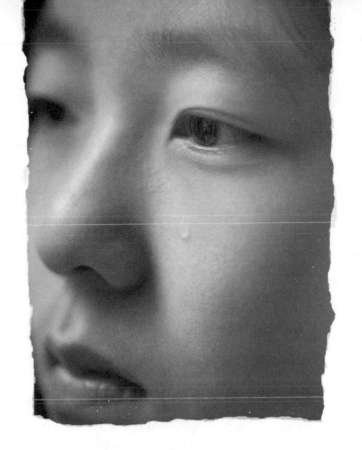

Chapter Five

Holding:
Creating a Safe Haven for the Patient
and Family

A [caregiver] helps a patient . . . by being lovingly present with that person; by being trustworthy, interested; and by believing that their joint activity will ultimately be redemptive and healing.

—IRWIN YALOM,
PHYSICIAN AND PROFESSOR OF PSYCHIATRY

Devotion. Moms learn about it, sometimes to their astonishment. It sneaks up on them. They may not know that it has become part of their being until a momentary brush with danger (real or imagined) brings it suddenly and sharply into focus. They will stop at nothing to protect their own child. They have officially become the "mama bear," claws out, ready to roar if the situation requires it.

For fathers it may take a different form. A dad may plan in advance just what to do as he walks down the street with his toddler, should an approaching stranger happen to have a gun or even just bad intentions. By the time they pass, the dad may already know which way he would have run, after he scooped up his little one, if the threat had materialized. He may continue to have fantasies about just how he would have pulverized the guy, had the guy made a move to harm his child.

Something rises up in us when they are at risk of harm, betrayal, or even gossip.

These are forms of devotion. Evolution may have put the feeling there, along with all the supporting biochemistry and neurology, but the actual experience of devotion in daily life is as tangible as any feeling a person will ever have. We want to defend the people to whom we are devoted. Something rises up in us when they are at risk of harm, betrayal, or even gossip. We want what is best for them and are prepared to make sacrifices to see that they get it.

Those to whom we are devoted are deeply affected by our stance toward them. Children whose parents were devoted to them are often strikingly secure, as if they somehow carry with them the idea that they are protected everywhere they go. Years later, such a child may act bravely on his own behalf when confronted with danger or anxiety. It's as if the parental devotion has invaded the child's body to become part of his makeup (Emde & Sorce, 1983; Main & Kaplan, 1985).

In sharp contrast, children whose parents were not devoted to them may be withdrawn and shy, full of irrational fears and wary of new situations or people. Or they may be full of bravado, trying to convince themselves and the world around them that they are tough and not as alone and defenseless as they actually feel. The awful lack of a sense of being protected has left them vulnerable; they want no one to see this reminder that no one was ever devoted to them (Trout, 1997; Trout, 2002).

We will see it in our patients, of course, since every last one of them was once a little child to whom someone was devoted— or to whom no one was devoted. A person who is ill often regresses, and old feelings of being safe and protected—or of being unsafe and unprotected—emerge (Strain, 1979). One patient will gladly put herself into our caring hands, imagining that she will be as safe with us as she was with a devoted parent years before. Another will hold us at great distance, devaluing our ministrations, fearful of vulnerability that will surely be followed by disappointment. Yet another will rage at us for not giving enough or not giving it fast enough, as she shadow-boxes the ghost of a parent who never showed up.

We will also see devotion in ourselves. Someone at the nurses' station is speaking unkindly about the patient in 307, and we find ourselves irritated, rising up to defend the one to whom we have mysteriously become devoted. We find ourselves pulled into a room, perhaps feeling drawn to sit and talk with a patient who is alone, even while the demands of the unit compel us to keep moving. We go the second mile with a family member or we take extra care to prepare a patient mentally, emotionally, and physically for transportation to another unit.

We make a phone call to check on the well-being of someone who remains in our mind long after discharge.

A pediatric nurse responds to a little boy's fearful question—"Am I going to die?"—with the surest sign of her devotion, and he knows her devotion is true: "Not on my watch!" It's a silly pledge, really; this nurse doesn't actually have the power over life and death that she has promised, but it doesn't matter. The message is received, and the little boy calms. Someone has his back. Someone has declared her devotion to him.

In health care, devotion seems to come with the territory. Even those of us with crusty exteriors know that it's still in there. It may be that devotion to others is in our nature; everybody knows it's our trademark. It's probably related to why we got into health care in the first place. Or maybe it's not in our nature at all; at least others wouldn't be quick to affirm that they see the trait in us. Still, a certain patient will bring it out, and there we are: protecting, defending, holding in our mind, looking after. We are saying by our presence, "I am completely here, and in my devotion to you, I will see to it that you are held."

A certain patient will bring it out, and there we are: protecting, defending, holding in our mind, looking after.

Holding Defined

Holding is an act of devotion. It's a conscious decision to lift up, affirm, and dignify that which the patient or family member has taught us, resulting in intense focus on the patient or family member while treasuring both the information and the person.

Like devotion, holding is almost never a one-time event. It is not a particular action, although action is most assuredly involved. It is a way of being with the patient that includes the characteristics of a fiercely-devoted parent. In daily practice, elements of holding expressed in action might include touch, but they also might include avoidance of touch—or exclusive use of a particular kind of touch—because that is what the patient has taught us he needs, and we have followed what he taught us.

If we have listened and if we have remembered, we know a great deal about what the patient wants. This listening to the patient, and remembering over time what he or she has said, are acts of holding.

Holding might also include steadfast refusal to join in on gossip or other idle and unfocused talk about the patient or family; we just feel too engaged with and protective of the patient or family member to disrespect them in this way. It might include a devotion to giving guidance to the hospitalist, the next nurse, the physical therapist, or the dietary aide, about how this patient's illness, or the dynamics around it, is likely to manifest in behavior; or what this patient's needs are with respect to food and eating; or what the main concerns of a family member are likely to be when he visits tonight; or what this patient is likely to be struggling with given the life she led before falling ill and coming to the hospital. We're not making assumptions nor conveying the information we've collected about the patient as though it were absolute. We're simply sharing what we know so that others might have a basis to ask even more meaningful questions, or to avoid touching what hurts or bringing up a painful subject in a way that doesn't respect the gravity of it for the patient.

Let's not make it complicated, though, and let's not assume we're talking about taking on extra duties in order to engage in holding.

Dr. Jill Bolte Taylor, the neuroanatomist we mentioned previously who wrote in 2006 about her massive left hemisphere stroke, described an interaction with one of her physicians this way:

> *Dr. David Greer was a kind and gentle young man. He was genuinely sympathetic to my situation and took the time to pause during his busy routine to lean down near my face and speak softly to me. He touched my arm to reassure me that I would be okay. Although I could not understand his words, it was clear to me that Dr. Greer was watching over me. He understood that I was not stupid but that I was impaired. He treated me with respect. I'll always be grateful for his kindness. (p. 75)*

So, can we develop a formula for holding? Can we make a list of the verbs subsumed under this strange-sounding practice in the therapeutic relationship? Dr. Greer "took the time"; he "leaned down"; he "touched"; he "watched over me"; he "understood"; he "treated me with respect." If we just do those things, will our patients experience holding? Perhaps they will.

But here's the dilemma: We are clinicians, not technicians. By definition, clinicians seek to know their patients by watching closely and gathering data. We convert our observations into diagnostic information and caregiving guidelines corresponding to what we've learned. It only worked for Dr. Greer to lean down near Dr. Bolte Taylor's face and speak softly to her because he understood something about what it might be like to have had a left hemisphere stroke. He knew her language comprehension would have been compromised, and her capacity for expressive language severely limited at least for the moment. He knew she would feel strangely distant from others (while wanting connection), might feel lonely, could probably still read social cues, and would be scared. He anticipated that one of her primary needs would be for human connection and reassurance about her safety. Dr. Greer found that he could easily provide both human connection and reassurance about her safety without investing extra time or stepping outside the boundaries of medicine.

Interestingly, the identical behaviors applied elsewhere might produce the opposite result. What if the patient had experienced a right hemisphere stroke instead? She might have been profoundly confused, perhaps even threatened, by social contact. Her needs might have been to "feed" the left side of her brain (now taking care of a greater load of the neurological business) that hungered for information, data, words, ideas, and the exercise of making logical connections between what had happened to her and the array of things that might happen next.

What if the patient were just in for a hernia repair, but a clinician saw those telltale signs that the patient had been sexually abused as a young girl (slight withdrawal from physical approach; slight flinching when touched; intense eye contact, as if wary and trying to collect information about the intentions of another; discomfort when too many residents or interns are in the room; or even an out-of-place seductiveness). Then some of Dr. Greer's behaviors, especially leaning down close, speaking softly, and touching the patient's arm, might well have been experienced as terrifying intrusions. This patient would not be held by these behaviors. She might best be held with much less physical proximity, interactions characterized by warm dignity, and lots of permission-asking, for example, "Who would you like to have in the room with you during your examination?"

Scripted behavior, by definition, cannot possibly take into consideration the uniqueness of every patient and every interaction. Rather, discernment is called for. Discernment is one of those characteristics for which nurses, physicians, therapists, and other clinicians are selected out of all the people in the world. Discernment is also something we have cultivated and consider to be one of our primary tools—sort of an invisible stethoscope.

This is not new information. We understand that we have something special, that we *do* something special. We use technology, and we have technical knowledge and acumen, but we are not technicians. We define ourselves instead as healers—or perhaps more accurately, as witnesses, co-conspirators in the service of healing.

It does take extraordinary concentration, devotion, and self-confidence to hold another. If we are skilled in attunement, it begins the moment we meet the person and begin to discover the illness. Rita Charon, professor of clinical medicine and director of the program in narrative medicine at Columbia University (2006) describes the initial meeting this way:

> I came to understand that what my patients paid me to do was to listen attentively to extraordinarily complicated narratives—told in words, gestures, silences, tracings, images, laboratory test results, and changes in the body—and to cohere all these stories into something that made provisional sense . . . . (p. 4)

Holding asks that we do these things:

- Holding asks us to pay attention; it means maintaining a therapeutic focus on the person.

- Holding asks us to remember in specific acts of care that which has been learned about the patient, the family, the culture, and the history, thus deeply complimenting the patient by recalling details that are important not only to diagnosis and treatment, but to the person.

- Holding asks us to carry the experience of the patient gently in our hands, keeping confidences as needed and appropriate, defending the patient against those who would disrespect her, lifting up her story as if it were our own.

- Holding means watching over the patient and family as a sentry, assuring their safety and the quality of their care.

- Holding means speaking of and writing about the patient and family—at change of shift report, in the hall, in notes—with dignity and an eagerness to transmit treasured information.

- Holding asks us to keep the patient and family informed about what is going on now and what is coming next.

- Holding asks us to be a steady and nonjudgmental presence in the face of the patient's physical suffering and strong emotional responses. We don't go away emotionally or physically.

- Holding asks us to demonstrate devotion to our patients and their families by creating a deeply collaborative relationship with our colleagues so that the patient and family experience being cared for by a dependable and interdependent health care team.

- Holding is guiding. Patients and their families are always at risk of feeling lost in the world of health care. We hold by providing information, by checking in often with patients and their family members to make sure that they are continually informed and continually included in the patient's care.

- Holding is offering informed reassurance— intentionally dissipating anxiety about an unknown by clarifying what is actually happening. Informed reassurance is based on the realities of the moment.

- Holding happens when clinicians who are attuned to the patient and family are devoted to wondering and following and to doing everything it takes to create a safe haven for the patient and family.

The meditation below, which Michael wrote for the *See Me As a Person* CD (Trout, 2011), recounts the power of a caring relationship between a patient and a nurse. The nurse, Ruth, cared in such a way that the person felt seen, safe, and whole.

Her Name Was Ruth

The first time she walked into my room, I knew.
She was to become, for me, like no other.

I had been around, as they say.
Chronic illness does that.
Health care people are in your life,
and in your face, all the time.

You start to notice differences.
Some can catch a vein on the first try, while others—
you just know it, before they even pick up the needle,
are going to stick you over and over,
and they're going to say, "Oops," and blame your arms for
having too-small veins
and forget completely that there's a person attached to
that arm.

Pretty soon you're noticing that others can't see so clearly:
the admitting clerks who, even by 7 a.m.,
are already so tired of sick people that they won't look you
in the eye.
But then there's the one who acts as if it really clicks
that the thing you are being admitted for is scaring you
to death.

The housekeeper for whom you are so completely
invisible,
lying there in that bed,
you might as well be a corpse.
But then there's the one for whom the act of mopping that
floor is an act of love.
As if they think their care of the floor is a way of caring
for you.
Which it is.

You notice the doctor who,
while talking to you about how she's going to stick her
hands into your chest
the next morning might as well be talking about making
some guacamole.
But then there's the one who catches on:
holding my heart is a great deal—like, well,
holding my heart.
For this doctor, it means something to hold another
human being's heart.
It isn't, for this special one, just about success rates.
This one knows that after tomorrow morning,
we will be connected forever.
Because she touched my heart.

You notice the nurses for whom we are more bodies than
people,
more workload than reasons-for-being.
For these, we exist only as "the PITA in 402,"
or the "frequent flyer" coming up from admitting.
But then there's the one who still remembers why she
became a nurse.
Which brings me back to Ruth, who gave me the gift
of sight.

Ruth, you see, saw me.
Every time she walked into my room, she would look at
me with new eyes.
I was not a problem.
I was not a gomer.
I was not a number.
I was a sick person, but I was also a whole person,
complete with a very big story
and lots of life behind me, and too little life in front
of me.

She saw my worry, and my dignity, and my smallness in
that bed,
and the bigness I used to have when I taught school and
raised my four kids.

I'll never know how she knew who I was and who I
might yet be.
Or why she stayed with me, in my sadness and my fear,
as they became smaller and softer.

I don't know how she did that.
How could one person's face communicate so much?
How could she get so much done without rushing,
and while making me feel as if I were not her problem,
but the very reason she got up today?

I told people who came to visit that I was safe.
Ruth was with me.
Her presence shone of safety
and warmth,
and strength.
It steadied me.

If this part is too weird, then just don't read it.
But I'm telling you there were moments when I saw my
tears in her eyes.

When Ruth was in the building, my earth was calm.
Somehow, those eyes of hers, that voice of hers, that touch
of hers
made me feel that she was sure about it all,
and that I could be too.

Much about this I don't understand.
All I can tell you is that Ruth—whose name I will never forget—
gave me the gift of sight.
Because Ruth, you see, saw me.

Bearing Witness to the Suffering of Another is Holding

Rita Charon, in her book, *Narrative Medicine: Honoring the Stories of Illness* (2006), reminds us that health care is continually re-humanized when caring physicians and nurses listen to the stories of their patients. She writes about narrative medicine as "medicine practiced with the skills of recognizing, absorbing, interpreting, and being moved by the stories of illness" (p. 4). These are the skills of a compassionate witness.

Charon stresses the importance of clinicians honoring the magnitude of the patient's experience by listening attentively, staying present, and bearing witness—often silent witness—to the suffering of that person. She asserts that it's witnessing that closes the divide that is so often experienced between patients and clinicians. These divides are related to the fear of mortality, and they're experienced by both patients and clinicians; they're triggered by the things we find difficult to look at, hard to be with. Much like Simone Weil, who reminded us that "the capacity to give one's attention to a sufferer is a rare and difficult thing" because of the vulnerability it stirs within us, Charon believes that these divides emerge as a protective wall that we construct when confronted with human emotions that make us feel vulnerable, such as shame, blame, and fear (p. 22).

Her description of bearing witness in the following interview excerpt (2007) invites clinicians to courageously cross the divide—even when they are not able to fix anything for the patient—and to simply be with the patient in his suffering:

Many of the outcomes that are measured cannot be separated from the importance of our ability to stay present with people in their suffering.

> *Bearing witness means letting another's suffering register on you. You recognize the suffering not for instrumental reasons of fixing it or doing something yourself in response to it...Our witness takes account of the gravity of that other person's lived experience. This is important for the health care professional because the posture conveys to the patient that the doctor or nurse grasps the gravity of the patient's situation and respects the magnitude of his or her plight. (p. 207)*

Charon points to a situation in which the caregiver truly can do nothing but care. The evidence of that caring as it's written on the clinician's face is an instrument of healing all on its own. In health care, we work in a culture of fast-paced doing. And in our results-oriented culture, our effectiveness is not measured in terms of how often we have served as silent witness to the suffering of another. We contend, however, that many of the outcomes that are measured cannot be separated from the importance of our ability to stay present with people in their suffering.

As we've already noted, it's a reality in health care that we are called to bear witness to sometimes repellent physical illnesses and injuries as well as the often hard-to-be-with emotions that our patients may be feeling. Sometimes we can help by doing, but sometimes there is nothing to be done other than to provide a sturdy presence, to be the person who stays both physically and emotionally present when the patient feels untouchable, unlovable, insufferable.

We know that this is one of those things you already do. We also know that it is among the most challenging things you do, and that when you do it your patients feel held. It is our aim that when you encounter moments in which there is nothing to do for your patients beyond the silent witnessing of their suffering, you remember that simply witnessing is, in fact, an act of healing.

Witnessing allows you to stay present, to let this person's suffering register on your face, to use touch to assure the patient that you're here, and perhaps to say, "I'm going to stay with you, and we're going to get through this together." The patient rests into the sturdiness of the clinician and feels held.

Holding Requires each Encounter to have a Beginning, Middle, and End

In the world of health care, the clinician is a tour guide in an often frightening foreign world. The clinician is the "native" in the clinical culture, and everyone who enters that culture will have a different understanding of it. The one commonality, however, is that those who don't already work within that culture are likely to experience it as foreign. Under ideal circumstances a person might bring a sense of adventure to delving into something foreign, but by definition, patients are not experiencing ideal circumstances. Instead, patients tend to feel uncertain and alone until the gap is closed between their own culture and the strange one they have entered.

Right from the outset, this culture gap creates a "hole" in the patient's experience of being held, and consciously or not, the patient feels the very real possibility of falling through that hole.

When we experience even a temporary dependency due to illness or trauma we feel vulnerable and powerless, so being "dropped" becomes a tangible concern. Clearly, our attuning, wondering, and following go a long way in creating the safe haven that patients depend upon for their sense of being held while they're in our care. In theory, there should be a cumulative effect of all of this conscious connection building that we're doing with our patients, but in practice, that connection and the sense of safety that goes with it can be undone in a moment. If, while you're away from your patient, he has a bad experience with a blood draw or a difficult interaction with another clinician or receives unexpected news delivered in a less-than-compassionate way, his world can be shaken to its foundations, and his experience of feeling safe and connected in your care may be undone.

It's clear from these examples that the patient's feeling of disorientation—of being lost in a foreign land—doesn't only happen for the patient at admission time; the admissions process is only one of many border crossings in the patient's experience. When we make sure that every interaction we are part of has a clear beginning, middle, and end, we continually re-orient the patient, which helps him to feel secure and held.

The Beginning: Meeting, Greeting, Orienting

Patients and families are continually dependent upon clinicians for reorientation to the moment. While the importance of clearly marking the beginning of a clinician-patient interaction is obvious when you meet the patient for the first time or during shift changes or when new clinicians enter the patient's life, it is just as important to clearly mark the beginning of all subsequent interactions, whether anything new is expected to happen or not.

This orientation is something that can and must happen continually, as patients and their families, once oriented to their surroundings and the generalities of their situations, cannot be expected to be oriented to new procedures or protocols nor to clinicians whom they have not yet met. However, even procedures and protocols that a patient may become familiar with over time are, in a sense, continually new. For example, the experience of presenting your arm for a blood draw the first time may be significantly different from the experience of presenting it for the third time in three days.

We all fail at times to mark our beginnings. In our day-to-day interactions with the people in our lives, we sometimes skip the niceties and cut to the chase. We do this with our friends and colleagues, with our own families, and unfortunately, we sometimes do it with our patients and their families.

It may be human nature (though perhaps greatly amplified in those who feel the pressures of time constraints) to want to launch directly into what one might consider the "actual work" to be done on behalf of the patient. If your aim is to clarify some historical data or administer medication or inform the person about an upcoming procedure, you might be tempted to begin describing your aim before pausing to say hello, making eye contact, or inquiring about the state of the person in order to help her prepare for your interaction. No matter what sort of task you're there to do, however, there's always some preparation to do with the person. It may be to help the patient manage the pain of a procedure, but it may also simply be to prepare her for what's coming—which in many cases means preparing her for what's about to be done to her or to a family member.

When the meeting, greeting, and orientation of a therapeutic beginning are skipped, it's likely that trust will be compromised and the patient's and family's anxiety and fear increased. These may become the people who are subsequently described as demanding or angry or uncooperative, when really they're just people who weren't given proper orientation to the moment. These now "demanding, angry, uncooperative" people were dropped—and they were dropped by us.

It is hoped that the practice of marking the beginning of each encounter with a greeting and a few highly-attuned moments of authentic relationship building will become second nature for every clinician.

It is hoped that the practice of marking the beginning of each encounter with a greeting and a few highly-attuned moments of authentic relationship building will become second nature for every clinician. This is where the practice of wondering can serve a clinician especially well. When we're truly interested in our patients we want to connect, and connecting as people at the beginning of every interaction sets the tone for everything that happens in that encounter. A disconnected beginning is hard to shift, but a beginning marked by our presence and attunement to where the patient seems to be physically, mentally, and emotionally, will set the tone for a clinical encounter in which the patient and family feel held.

The Middle: Collaborating, Intervening, Deepening

The middle phase is the one in which the functional purpose for the interaction is carried out. If in this phase the clinician is rushed or distracted, the connection is diminished. If the clinician is present, attuned, curious, and caring, the connection is deepened and trust grows.

Connection can be deepened in the middle phase of the therapeutic relationship through actions such as:

- reassuring the patient during procedures,

- preparing the patient adequately for physical pain,

- asking permission to touch the patient,

- validating the patient's reports about his or her own body, and

- inviting family members to be aware of procedures when appropriate.

These caring actions are supported by our remembering to honor the dignity and experience of each patient and each patient's loved ones, and by a practice built on the belief that such connection facilitates improved healing and health.

The middle phase is also a time in which it can be demonstrated that clinicians are working closely with each other and appropriately sharing information about patients. If a patient is asked numerous questions at admission and then subsequent clinicians use that information in their interactions with the patient and family, it demonstrates several things to the patient and family that they may be aware of consciously or perhaps only subconsciously. Efficient transmission of information about the patient between clinicians demonstrates: 1) that clinicians are connected to each other and are interested in incorporating important information about the patient; 2) that the energy exerted by the patient and family in providing the information is respected and therefore the information is used and communicated between members of the team; and 3) that systems within the organization are coordinated, efficient, thoughtful, and designed to provide a satisfying experience for the patient and family.

In the absence of visible collaboration, coordination, and efficient systems, patients and their families are likely to feel weary, impatient, dissatisfied, mistrustful, and dropped.

The End: Transitioning, Supporting, Preparing

When patients are engaged in any sort of transition, they are at the greatest risk for feeling dropped. This doesn't just refer to the transition that occurs at the end of a patient's hospital stay, emergency room visit, or clinic appointment. Every clinical interaction includes a transition, and there are countless reasons to tend to them carefully.

In all clinical settings, especially hospitals, patients are continually at risk for feeling disoriented as any sort of transition occurs. Patients may not know what to expect next, and they may not know what's expected of them. When they are left not knowing, they may feel abandoned and fearful. However, when transitions are managed artfully, with the patient and family being fully involved and informed, care is experienced as seamless and is understood by all.

Figure 5.1 below illustrates the recursive three-phase process of clinical encounters.

FIGURE 5.1: The Three Phases of a Therapeutic Interaction

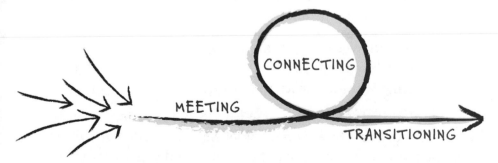

It's important to note that these three phases do not describe what happens automatically within a clinician-patient encounter. Instead they comprise a conscious three-step framework that, when put into action, helps the patient to feel held. It becomes important to shine a light on these phases because in chaotic, fast-paced environments it's human nature to want to go directly to the task at hand, sometimes forgetting the importance of meeting and transitioning patients. While this framework could appear to take more time, in the long run time is saved. Those who are well prepared for what's coming next are less likely to become angry, frustrated, anxious, high-demand patients and families.

Imagine yourself in the role of patient or family member under these circumstances:

- A new nurse arrives to care for you and you didn't realize your other nurse had left; there was no preparation or transition between this nurse and the previous one.

- A new physician is suddenly involved in the care of your father, and the primary physician didn't let you know this physician's consultation had been requested or that she would be stopping in.

- You are surprised when a transport aid arrives to take you to a procedure without preparation or information from the clinicians caring for you about why it was scheduled or what is to be done to you.

- You discover that you are scheduled for an invasive procedure only when you learn that your breakfast is being held until after the procedure.

You wonder if this new nurse knows what is important to you; you wonder why this new physician was called and what she understands about your father; you wonder if you want to have this test or procedure done and why you weren't involved in the decision. The result is that, as the patient or the family member supporting the patient, you may feel that you are the last to know and that you are there to be "done to" rather than playing an integral part in your own care or the care of your loved one. Experiences such as these shake trust and can create a sense of isolation. This *doing to* rather than *collaborating with* a patient does not happen because caregivers are disrespectful or malicious; it is, however, a risk in high-volume, fast-paced environments in which clinical staff have ever-shifting responsibilities.

If we remember how important each phase is to the person receiving care we will use the framework to help us remember to slow down and pay attention to how we might build, deepen, and preserve our relationships with our patients and their families throughout each phase.

Holding in Times of Crisis

During the 2010 NCAA basketball Final Four game between West Virginia University (WVU) and Duke University, WVU's Da'Sean Butler drove to the basket and straight into Duke's monster center Brian Zoubek. Their knees crashed together, and Butler dropped to the floor writhing in pain. The game was halted for several minutes because Butler could not get up; he had suffered a torn anterior cruciate ligament (ACL) and sprained his medial collateral ligament (MCL). The team physician examined him, and then WVU coach Bob Huggins—a bear of a man himself—strode over to his star player.

To everyone's astonishment, Coach Huggins got down on all fours, kneeling over this young man whom he was now treating like a son. Butler, without a thought to his own pain, started apologizing, distressed only that his injury might jeopardize his team's chances at the national championship that he wanted so badly for his coach to have. "Coach, I'm sorry I couldn't get you your first national championship," he said through his tears.

Huggins responded by cradling Butler's head in his hands, looking him straight in the eye, his nose only inches from Butler's, and saying, "Don't worry about it. You're a special kid," and then, "I love you" (CBS Sports, 2010, April 3).

In interviews later, this wounded warrior said that the coach's words calmed him down and that he would remember the moment for the rest of his life (Larry Brown Sports, 2010, April 6).

This is holding. It was literal holding, of course: a big man cradling a young athlete in his arms and calming him with his resolute presence and tender words. It was also, it its way, the sort of holding about which we speak in this chapter: a leader exercises his authority to create a tender circle around a person in excruciating physical and emotional pain, assuring him, putting him before all else. Nothing mattered at that moment except an athlete's agony and a coach's empathy. We imagine Da'Sean Butler will pay it forward someday. It's what happens when we feel truly and fully held. We remember the feeling forever, and we want others to have it too.

A distinction must be made, of course, between the sort of holding that can comfortably take place between two people in a personal relationship and what can and should happen within the therapeutic relationship. Huggins and Butler knew each other well and had forged a father-son bond that inspired Huggins to act as he did and Butler to respond accordingly.

There is, however, a version of holding in crisis situations within the therapeutic relationship that approximates what happened between Huggins and Butler. There is no question that holding in a crisis is different from holding in the lower-impact day-to-day realities of

In a crisis, time feels different. The dynamic of leader-and-led stays the same, but everything appears to speed up.

the clinician-patient relationship, but the dynamic of 1) the compassionate, knowledgeable, experienced leader, and 2) the person who is in pain, unsure, and temporarily starved for reassurance, is a dynamic that shows up in even the most routine therapeutic encounter.

In a crisis, time feels different. The dynamic of leader-and-led stays the same, but everything appears to speed up. In crisis situations we become keenly aware of the actions we must take in order to assist the person in immediate need. For most of us, whether we physically speed up or not, a switch flips, and suddenly our level of alertness increases, a number of chemical reactions are triggered in our brains, and those chemicals quickly begin to flood our bodies.

In these crisis situations, our words become more important than ever. It isn't so much that the pressure is on us to say just the right thing at just the right time. Instead, it becomes more important than ever for our words to reflect a high level of attunement with our patients as well as to convey information that is highly relevant. For example, "Everything's going to be just fine," may be adequate reassurance when one is not in crisis, but when pain is acute and mounting steadily, the patient would much rather hear, "I've given you some medication in your IV; your pain will begin to ease significantly in just a few seconds."

Interestingly, even in crisis situations holding is still created and nurtured by the clinician's careful tending to the distinct beginning, middle, and end of the therapeutic encounter. It would seem that emergencies would constitute the one time that the patient actually benefits from our getting right to the administration of care—jumping right to the middle, as it were. However, abundant anecdotal evidence indicates that the opposite is true. We consistently hear that the most satisfying patient-clinician emergency encounters begin with an introduction and orientation for the patient (regardless of whether he or she is conscious). EMTs and other emergency clinicians routinely tell the patient their name and role, make an attempt to establish the patient's name as well as getting other information from the patient, and provide the patient with information about the state of his or her condition as well as what care is being administered. The middle of the encounter is marked by administration of care and informed reassurance, and the end is marked by a transfer of information about the patient to the clinician who will take over once the emergency responder is out of the picture. In the most satisfying of these encounters the patient is introduced to the new clinicians (when possible) and they immediately begin orienting the patient to the new setting and care team. Could it be that crisis situations bring out the intuitive holder in most of us? Is it actually easier to be thorough in a fast-paced setting than it is in a less acute setting?

Whether that's the case or not, at the very least we can see that holding doesn't have to take any more time than does failing to hold. When clinicians ask questions and share information freely and perhaps routinely (in the best sense of the word) it only makes sense that patients are then more likely to feel oriented and less likely to become dissatisfied with their care.

The consideration of holding in crisis situations gives us one more lens through which to look at how holding does or doesn't show up in our own daily practice. Once you begin to notice holding (and perhaps also its opposite: dropping), you'll see that there are times when holding is challenging to do and times when it's nearly automatic. Sometimes it's masterful and elegant, and indeed sometimes it's clumsy and awkward, though perhaps no less effective in its unrefined form. When your words, affect, and actions all say, "I'm here for you," in even the smallest way, you're holding the patient, and the patient feels it and becomes more secure within it, whether he consciously notices it or not.

Holding in the Face of Anger

It's a tough spot to be in, isn't it? Suddenly, right in the middle of an interaction with someone for whom we are caring, there are fireworks. We're on the receiving end of somebody's anger, and it seems mighty personal. We want to hold this patient—indeed we thought we were—and now it has blown up. The provision of care under these circumstances is challenging to say the least. Even maintaining professional dignity is tough.

Michael sometimes works with children who urinate on things such as laundry, restaurant windows, or pets. They have volcanic, fire-breathing anger. Because he's privy to the history of these children, it takes little imagination for him to know that the rage is not at the dirty clothes.

Even when the anger erupts as an expletive-spitting, demeaning, withering volley of words directed at the beleaguered foster mother who has done nothing more than set a modest limit, we know that it is the original mother (the one who abused him and then threw him away or who failed to protect him from another abuser) who is the real target. The foster mother is a mere stand-in for the one who hurt him.

This sort of anger comes from frustration, from fear, from vulnerability and from hating vulnerability, from intolerable impotence—converted in the moment into an attempt to take charge (Hughes, 2007; Keck & Kupecky, 1995; Levy & Orlans, 1998; Pruett, 1984; Trout & Thomas, 2005). In these ways, our angry patients or their angry families resemble these hurt children.

It is essential for us to remember that the target is not us.

In these moments, it becomes essential for us to remember that the target is not us. The target is the vulnerability created by illness, the feeling of impotence created by crippling conditions. The target is systems that won't/can't/don't make the patient feel safe. The target is a ghost: a father who humiliated the patient many years ago and who now metaphorically comes back to visit in the form of a situation that makes the patient again feel small and helpless.

It feels like the anger is being aimed at us, of course. After all, we are the recipients of the monumental, irrational rage right there in the moment, in front of everybody. But that's why we told you about the children. If we respond to these rage-filled children in foster care by taking personally what they say and do to us, we're sunk. We can't help. Our empathy shuts down, and all we can think about is defending ourselves. It is natural to feel defensive when it appears that we're being attacked unless we are somehow able to re-frame, to remember where this steaming ball of venom came from, and to recall the origins of the awful energy this child is hurling at us.

And here's an irony that may allow the metaphor to help us even further: The best response to such fury in little foster children is to pick them up, hold them close, and repeat, "I know, sweetheart. Your heart is breaking. I know. You feel so helpless. I'm sorry. I'm here" (Becker-Weidman & Shell, 2010; Hughes, 2009).

"What?!"—responds any sensible layperson to such bizarre advice about how to respond to outbursts from abused children in foster care, but it's true. The thing that breaks through the attack from such an overwhelmed little one is not a lecture ("Now young man; that's no way to talk!"), or a consequence (for what? for having been abused and being ticked off about it now?), and certainly not a verbal retort ("I can yell louder than you can!").

The thing that breaks through the attack is holding.

For the first few seconds, of course, holding is not welcomed. After all, being held when one is angry increases feelings of vulnerability. But that is the point: The child is vulnerable; he can't run things; you are in charge. He will have to live with that. What parents can offer is their almost unbearable comfort. If the child can accept it (and he almost invariably can after much hesitation), he will have a much better chance of getting through life with less rage, more empathy, less demandingness, and more openness (Hughes, 2007; Levy & Orlans, 1998).

While we may not collect the patient or family member in our arms (at least that's not the only way to make people feel held), we can hold in countless other ways.

- We can listen without defense or retort.

- We can be curious.

- We can let the person know she is seen and heard and maybe even understood.

- We can say, "I'm sorry"—not as an acknowledgement of our own culpability, but as a way to communicate that we "get" that she feels wronged or ignored.

- We can touch with our eyes as well as with our fingertips.

We can say with our posture, with our touch, with our unwavering presence: I am interested in you; I am with you; I am here.

Holding is Creating a Safe Haven for the Patient

In this section we share two stories illustrating the effects that a health care team's connectedness or lack of connectedness can have on patients' sense of being held. The first story was told to us by the mother of a young adolescent girl who suffers with a chronic illness.

Connection Creates Comfort

Following a rather routine outpatient surgery my daughter Jenny began to experience severe headache and flushing. It was extremely frightening, as the pain seemed to be increasing steadily. The attending nurse assessed Jenny and decided to contact the surgeon and let him know what was happening. The surgeon said he would come in immediately.

In the meantime, the nurse remained with us, talking with Jenny, placing some cold packs on her body. She asked Jenny if she could rub her feet, suggesting that, strangely enough, pressure on her feet may help ease the pain in her head. Jenny agreed and the nurse gently uncovered her feet and massaged them while she continued to speak reassuringly to Jenny. She let us know that the doctor was on his way and would be able to evaluate what was going on.

"It's likely," the nurse said, "that you're reacting to the anesthesia and perhaps the morphine. When the doctor determines exactly what it is, he'll be able to take care of it." All this while the nurse was touching Jenny's feet at pressure points and with gentle massage. Even though Jenny's pain continued, her fear— which at one point had reached near-panic levels—diminished.

Within what seemed to both Jenny and me like only minutes, the surgeon arrived and diagnosed that Jenny was in adrenal crisis, and he asked the nurse to administer corticosteroids in intravenous fluid. Jenny's symptoms began to ease. The surgeon's swift action resolved the crisis, and the nurse's gentle attendance and astute initial assessment helped Jenny cope with the crisis and made sure the right action was taken.

Before the surgeon left the room, he turned to young Jenny and extended his hand. Jenny shook his hand as he said to her, "You're doing fine now... agree?" Jenny nodded. "I'm confident you're going to continue to recover without a problem now, but if anything at all is of concern, your nurse will contact me immediately." He squeezed her hand and then turned to the nurse and extended his hand to her. The nurse shook it as he said to her, "Thank you. Your assessment and speedy response is why Jenny is going to be just fine. I appreciate working with you, Alice. I always know our patients are in good hands when you're here."

Because of Jenny's illness we'd spent a lot of time in hospitals and we'd worked with many teams, but I'd never seen anything like the level of professional connection these two colleagues had with each other. Their visible respect and teamwork made me feel that Jenny was safe in their care and allowed me to rest more easily that night.

What does Jenny get from this interaction? What does her mother get? First, both the nurse and the surgeon touched, cared for, and held Jenny with competence and compassion. Then, when the surgeon visibly acknowledged the nurse in front of Jenny and her mother, his expression of esteem for the nurse created an even deeper sense of safety for both of them. When they saw such clear evidence that Jenny's physician and nurse were there for each other, they knew they could count on the team to continue to hold her through the night.

When clinicians visibly hold each other in high esteem, the patient's sense of security increases.

Can we conclude that such visible teamwork is a therapeutic intervention in and of itself? Could it be that when clinicians visibly hold each other in high esteem, the patient's sense of security increases?

Now contrast Jenny's story with a story contributed by the mother of an adult daughter who also suffers from a chronic disease. As she is admitted to an emergency department for treatment, her care team is far less connected than the team caring for Jenny.

If the Team is Disconnected, the Patient Feels Lost

Tina was in terrible pain after infusion of intravenous immunoglobulin (IVIG) for rejection of her transplanted kidney. Her head pounded, her joints ached so much that she couldn't sleep at night even with medication, and the pain didn't subside in the days following her treatment. Five days after her treatment she called the oncologist who was overseeing her IVIG and he told her to go to the emergency room. She called me reluctantly, because she doesn't like to worry me; if Tina called, I knew it was serious.

When I got there, Tina and her fiancé were already there talking with the triage nurse. In the ER, I could see all kinds of plaques and posters saying things like "Ask us anything," "We care about you," and "We want to do our best for you."

The triage nurse had her brow pinched as she asked Tina questions in a flat tone of voice, asking often for information to be repeated, entering the data as quickly as she could, and facing the computer instead of Tina the whole time.

As I walked in, Tina was going through all her medications with the nurse who appeared bored and detached even though the lengthy list of medications suggested a serious chronic condition. She didn't show any interest at all in this young woman who was managing (or possibly mismanaging, for all she knew) such a serious chronic illness. The nurse asked Tina several times to repeat information as she worked to complete the admission documentation. When she finally got all the information, the nurse said, barely looking at Tina, "Okay sweetie, you can go to your room now . . . . we're putting you in the critical care room because you're immunosuppressed, but if a real crisis comes in you will be moved out. " She walked ahead of Tina to the room and put a gown on the table. "Your nurse should be in soon." She walked out without glancing at Tina.

Once we got to the room, a very friendly nurse came in and introduced herself. She made good eye contact and had a very caring manner, but it soon became clear, as this nurse asked a lot of the same questions again, that none of the information from Tina's arduous admission had made it past the triage desk. I did my best to stay in the background as my blood began to boil. This nurse could see that Tina was in pain, and every inefficiency was flashing in front of me like a neon sign because all I wanted in the world was for somebody to help relieve my daughter's pain and figure out what was wrong with her. Ironically, just as I was having that thought, I heard someone in the hall say, "I don't have time for this." My dander was up and I thought, *It's no wonder you don't have time. Take a look at how you're* using *your time! Right now, in front of me, someone is duplicating the exact same process my daughter was subjected to five minutes ago.* This nurse's demeanor was sweet and accommodating, but her manner did not make up for the impression that she was neither prepared nor connected with others on the team.

The ER doctor came in and was also very friendly. However, he greeted Tina with, "So, what brings you in this morning?"

Tina paused before she spoke because she thought he might be joking; she had told two nurses in agonizing detail why she was here. Certainly they must have passed that information on? But it seemed that they had not. The doctor was serious; he did not know why she was in the department or anything about her complicated history. At this point, I started to worry that he might not even know what it meant that she was a transplant patient or what it meant to be receiving IVIG treatment for rejection, nor why she was having such a severe reaction to the infusion she had days ago (if that was in fact the problem). I asked what he knew about the side effects of IVIG.

At that point he assured us he would be talking with Tina's oncologist.

We were somewhat eased by that information because with all of the disconnections in communication we were becoming quite terrified. There was no sense of continuity. Each clinician started from scratch. Because of their discon-nected approach, we did not feel like Tina was in safe and competent hands. Because my daughter was vulnerable and in pain, I felt I had to stay close and be extremely vigilant in order to keep her safe.

This team was not a team. There was no visible in-fighting, and it's possible that morale on the unit was perfectly fine, but there was also no teamwork; they functioned as parallel players rather than interdependent team members. It was clear to the patient and family that the clinicians were either not sharing information or not trusting each other's ability to collect and record the patient's information correctly.

It might seem that a team's lack of connection is something patients and their families wouldn't be aware of, at least in the absence of actual conflict. In fact, it may be true that a patient and family might not be able to put their finger on what it is that is making them feel dropped in our care, but they do, nonetheless, feel dropped.

The electronic health record (EHR) is a great adjunct to care if it's used as one. Tina's emergency room visit could have gone differently had the EHR been used in this way. What would it have meant to this patient's experience had Nurse 2 looked at the documentation that Nurse 1 had so arduously collected? She still could have confirmed and clarified the information, but there would have been some continuity, and perhaps most importantly, the time between Tina's walking in the door and having some relief for the pain she'd been suffering with for five days would have been shorter and less frustrating. Tina would have felt like the time in triage was an important investment in her receiving care. What if the triage nurse had attuned to Tina and let her know that she understood how uncomfortable Tina was? What if she reassured Tina that she was asking so many questions in order to be thorough and so that the rest of the team would be prepared for her? What if the assigned nurse who introduced herself so pleasantly and made such good eye contact with Tina had familiarized herself with what the first nurse had documented and began with, "Now here's what I'm understanding is going on . . . " rather than starting cold, repeating the process, exacerbating Tina's misery, and frustrating her family? What if the assigned nurse and physician had collaborated prior to the physician entering Tina's room, so that he could build on the information gathered and strengthen the care and connection with Tina?

Holding the Patient's Family as Part of the Safe Haven

Some patients' family members define their role as advocate for their loved one's care while others simply try to buffer the harsh effects of an unfamiliar environment while their loved one is vulnerable. Worried, uprooted from their own routines, family members may need holding and assurance of safety just as much or more than the patient does. Here is a story from Mary's own experience about being held in safe haven as a family member:

Commitment to Care for Families

In 1990, a mere six months following my father's death from Alzheimer's, I received a phone call in the middle of the day from the emergency department at St Peter's Hospital in Olympia, Washington. The person on the line informed me that my mother had been taken by ambulance to the emergency room and her physician would like to talk with me. The cardiologist told me that my mother had been rushed to the hospital after suffering a massive cardiac arrest. He assured me that EMTs had arrived immediately upon call and everything possible was being done to save my mother's life. This sort of news is always dreadful, and on top of having just lost my father, it was almost more than I could bear. I took the next flight out of Minneapolis to Seattle, not knowing whether my mother would be alive when I arrived at St Peter's. I was somewhat comforted by the words of the cardiologist as he spoke with me on the phone. He was compassionate and honest. He did not know whether Mom would make it, but his calm reassurance and comprehensive information inspired trust in me and I believed everything possible was being done to save my mother.

When I arrived on the critical care unit, I was met by a nurse who asked if I was Ms. Koloroutis' daughter and said they had been expecting me. She put her arm around my shoulder as my knees shook, and said she could imagine how frightening this was for me, especially with my having been so far away, but that she wanted me to know that my mother was stable and that there was growing optimism that she would be able to pull through. The nurse asked if I was prepared to see my mom on a respirator. I was grateful for her kindness and for her preparation.

As I entered my mother's room, the nurse caring for her came to the door to greet me. "I am so glad you're here. Your mom is holding on. She must be quite a lady! I can see her strength. Let me tell you what has happened so far and what all of the equipment and medications are for..." With that, mom's attending nurse covered all that was happening in a calm and thorough manner. The nurse then called the cardiologist; he wanted to know when I arrived so he could come by and talk with our family about my mother's care and recovery. He arrived within the hour and sat with my brothers and me to let us know precisely what had transpired and what we could expect in the next 24 hours, and he reassured us that the whole team was watching over Mom and that things were progressing very well. My brothers and I began to breathe easier and believe that Mom and all of us who loved her would get through this.

That night, I slept at my mother's home. I did not hold vigil in the waiting room or inside my mother's room. I trusted that she was being watched over, and I knew I could come in or call at any time. Her nurse had told me just that, and it was clear to me that the health care team and our family were in this together

More than twenty years later, this experience is etched in my mind and heart. I felt held in the competence, confidence, compassion, and presence of the caregivers. I remember noticing a poster by the central station on the unit. I cannot recall these many years later exactly what it said. What I do remember was that it was a statement of commitment to care for the families of the patients on the critical care unit.

This story demonstrates what it means to hold the patient and the family in the center of our care. All three phases of the therapeutic relationship were deftly attended to in this story. The nurse was expecting Mary and even greeted her by name. The cardiologist followed shortly, and Mary found that he was also aware of what deep distress she was likely to be in, given both her mother's condition and the recent passing of her father. Then the nurse, who may even have known that Mary "spoke fluent hospital" under normal circumstances, correctly surmised that she might very well require just as much orientation as anyone else to the foreign land of that exact medical setting under those exact circumstances. The nurse and physician kept Mary informed about what was happening as it happened and prepared her for what was happening next in her mother's care.

When common ground is found, we are able to empathize with the experiences of patients and families so thoroughly that we actively see every patient interaction as a shared human experience.

In this story, Mary and her family felt as though they'd been shepherded through their experience by people who wondered about what this experience meant for them, listened to what they said (and didn't say), and made sure that Mary and her family knew that the staff was watching over her mother. Trust was easy for them because it was so obvious that their experience mattered deeply to their caregivers—it was clear that common ground was established. The caregivers offered their expertise along with their presence and concern, so that the experience of Mary's mother's illness would be as easy as possible for the family.

Common ground is established when caregivers make the choice to "care deeply" for patients and to cultivate a relationship of trust and emotional safety (Sanghavi, 2006, p. 288). When common ground is found, we are able to empathize with the experiences of patients and families so thoroughly that we actively see every patient interaction as a shared human experience. It's not "this is you being sick, and this is me caring for you." Instead, it's what the entire team at St. Peter's said to Mary, though sometimes with their actions rather than their words: "We are in this together." A culture in which seeking and finding common ground are the norm allows for a way of interacting in which we integrate and consistently demonstrate that we as human beings are universally connected. Trust is easy in such a culture of connection.

The understanding that our need for care is a universal human need—that the "stretcher" is indeed a great equalizer—is solidly understood and consistently demonstrated in caregivers who seek common ground.

It is also essential to note that the culture of connection in the St. Peter's ICU is ultimately a culture that is intentionally created, and there is infrastructure in place to support it. It's a culture that requires both the therapeutic presence of each clinician and a level of support within the health care team that continually encourages caregivers—as the therapeutic relationship requires—to wonder, follow, and hold every patient and every family in their care. While it is always possible for an individual clinician to practice wondering, following, and holding, the degree of holding evident in Mary's story is one that depends upon an entire team for its creation and sustenance.

We ask you now to consider a story that is vastly different from the story Mary tells about her mother's hospitalization in Olympia. It is a true story and was contributed in hopes that it would help improve the care of others in similar circumstances.

"They're Treating My Father Like He's a Lump in the Bed"

Laura's voice on the other end of the phone sounded exhausted, and she was fighting tears. Her father had suffered a massive stroke while in the hospital for what was expected to be a routine surgical procedure. Halfway through the surgery, she and her family were told, in a matter-of-fact (and they thought defensive) way, that their father had suffered a stroke and that it was not because of the surgery. From that moment on the family were struck by the seemingly rote manner of the care their father received; it appeared that people were tending only to the physical needs of a body. Nobody on the hospital staff initiated support for them, and they were left to speculate that the care team just wanted their father to be gone so they could forget about this episode.

The family was devastated by his stroke. They were reeling from this traumatic loss of the father as they knew him. He was a powerful, exuberant man—their primary provider—who had always been able to make things right. In an instant, that had all changed; he couldn't speak or move. He was completely vulnerable, dependent on others for almost everything. Laura and her family were bewildered and afraid. The world as they knew it had stopped. The father they knew was gone.

In one attempt to connect with the family, a nurse who was handling their father rather roughly asked a member of the family, "What did your dad do for a living?" They said he was a realtor. The nurse then said that she'd had terrible experiences with realtors—"they do so little for their money; it's ridiculous that they should walk away with such a high percentage of the sale..."

It was then that Laura called a nurse friend for help. She wanted to know how to get her father's nurse taken off his care. As her friend instructed, she went to the nurse manager and said they didn't feel safe and that they didn't want this nurse caring for their father. Later that day, the nurse confronted Laura about talking to her manager. The family assumed that after that event they would be labeled as a difficult family and they felt even further isolated. Laura wasn't asking for sophisticated medical interventions. She was pleading for basic kindness and respect for her father as a person needing care.

She wanted the nurses to stop talking over him and instead to talk softly to him. She wanted the transport team to stop moving him roughly and hurriedly and instead touch him gently and move him with care. The family had no reason to assume that he wasn't getting all of the right medications and the appropriate medical follow-through. What was missing was the appropriate therapeutic care for both him and the family. What was missing was the creation of an environment in which it would at least be possible for them all to begin healing both emotionally and physically.

She asked her nurse friend, "Do they know something I don't know? Can he not hear or feel anything? Isn't he still here? Doesn't he deserve basic human kindness and dignity?"

This intense feeling of disruption is a predictable human response for families of victims of stroke and other sudden and traumatic events. The patient and his loved ones have difficulty coping with a disorienting new reality in the face of extreme loss. The patient suffers a sense of discontinuity of the self and fears he will never be a whole person again. His family members fear that as well. The reality is that his wholeness will be redefined. The experience is described by stroke survivors as dark, lonely, and terrifying (Bolte Taylor, 2006; Engel, 2010; Thomas & Pollio, 2002).

For this family, to make matters worse, it was clear to them that their extremely vulnerable father was now at the mercy of a care team that seemed to care little about him. Their discomfort grew steadily as they continued to witness what was for them an incredible incongruence between the magnitude of their own experience and the world of the care team. They had just experienced a life-altering tragedy, but the care team was going about their normal business in a way that suggested they weren't attuned at all to the meaning of this for the patient and family.

This family was yearning for some acknowledgement of their trauma, some sense of connection between themselves and the clinicians who were there, they thought, to take compassionate care of, if not them, at least their father. Instead, their reality and the reality of the health care team seemed worlds apart. On the walls of this unit, a sign announced that the hospital was a proud recipient of an award in recognition for excellence in nursing care. The hospital is also renowned for excellence in medical care. Laura knew that having taken her father to a hospital that had received such prestigious recognition meant that it was reasonable for her to expect to be guided and supported through this crisis by knowledgeable professionals who would understand the enormity of this episode in their lives while caring tenderly for her father. Instead, in the midst of the proclamations of excellence, Laura and her family felt isolated and alone in their suffering and afraid to leave their father's side. Their trust was shattered. They felt abandoned. Their healing was compromised.

When one member is suffering, the whole group suffers. When one relationship is ailing, all relationships are damaged. When one part of the whole feels less than a part, there is no whole anymore.

It's impossible to know for certain what was going on in the minds of the clinicians in this story, but it is certain that the family experienced being dropped rather than held. As the family suffered, the clinicians seemed to turn away from them, forgetting a principle that we hold dear: When one member is suffering, the whole group suffers. When one relationship is ailing, all relationships are damaged. When one part of the whole feels less than a part, there is no whole anymore (Trout, 1993).

When trust is compromised and people feel isolated and alone, they begin to make up their own stories. They begin to speculate about the thoughts and motives of the "others," deepening the divide even more, making common ground impossible. Since the patient's family had so little meaningful interaction with their father's caregivers, they even wondered if they were being rejected because something unexpected had happened during their father's surgery. Laura wondered, "Did that make them afraid of us?"

The reality is that family members are often the "co-authors" of the patient's experience; therefore, the family's perception of the patient's care matters. Family members are in the unique position of being intimately involved in the small details of the patient's care, while also seeing the big picture in ways that patients and clinicians do not. Consider this scenario: A patient is overjoyed by the standard of care he's receiving and is struck by the fact that human kindness seems to be a value that the care team holds dear . . . until his wife comes into his room and tells a story about how she overheard a physician on the phone speaking angrily to whomever happened to be on the other end of the line. The family member's experience in the hallway has suddenly become part of the patient's experience as well.

When patient satisfaction surveys are filled out, family members are often involved and may even be driving that process. Given this reality, from a business standpoint alone, we're putting our organizations at risk when we fail to care for the families of our patients. The truth is that the patient's experience is profoundly dependent on the family's experience. It's up to us whether we find this truth troublesome or we instead seize the opportunity it presents for us to provide a more satisfying care experience for our patients and their families.

Three Principles for Holding the Family

In well-respected care models such as Patient and Family-Centered Care, The Planetree Model, and Relationship-Based Care, *family* is understood to mean whomever patients identify as significant to them and their care. The degree of the family's involvement is determined by the patient if he is developmentally mature and competent (Frampton, Gilpin, & Charmel, 2003; Koloroutis, 2004; Kovasca, Bellin, & Fauria, 2006).

The degree of dependence the patient has on her family will vary significantly. However, irrespective of the degree of actual dependence, the influence of the family connection is a near constant in our patients' lives. To some clinicians, this is a rather frustrating reality. According to Frampton, Gilpin, and Charmel of the Planetree Group (2003), "When hospital staff members are asked to list the attributes of the 'perfect patient and family,' their response is usually 'a passive patient with no family'" (p. 54), and they describe the ideal patient this way:

- one who does not ask questions;

- one who never rings the call bell;

- one who does exactly what he or she is told; and

- one who has no visible family members or friends to advocate on his or her behalf.

In hospitals where this mindset prevails, families experience being treated more as "intruders than as loved ones . . . at best they are visitors. But, who are the real visitors in the patient's life—the staff of the hospital or the patient's family and friends?" (Frampton, Gilpin, & Charmel, 2003, p. 54).

While we recognize that not all families are equally willing or able to care for a family member, they are still the constant in the person's life; it is the health care team who are the transient visitors. Therefore it is in everyone's best interest for clinicians to cultivate authentic relationships with the family in order to maximize their ability to care for and support their loved one and to enhance the quality and safety of aftercare.

In order to better understand how we can hold our patient's family—the people who play such a vital role in our patient's healing—we'd like to introduce three principles for holding the family:

1. See the patient's family members as people needing our care and support.

2. See the patient's family members as essential members of the health care team.

3. Overcome obstacles to involving the family in the care of the patient by building on their strengths while respecting the differences in their relationships, coping methods, and individual circumstances.

When the practice of holding finds its most artful expression, and these three principles are attended to, a sense of security is created for the patient and family.

Seeing Family Members as People Needing Our Care and Support

When illness or trauma strikes one member of a family system, other members are affected in ways specific to their unique relationship with the patient. There are times, of course, when family members will rush to let you know how they're affected by the health crisis at hand. Other times they won't. In fact, they won't always know or fully understand the ways in which they're affected by their loved one's health crisis until they're well into it (if ever). That means we're called upon to care for people who may have no idea what they need in order to feel better.

Fortunately, as their guides in the foreign land of health care, we can offer them a number of things that have consistently proven effective in holding the patient's family:

- Authentically acknowledge how difficult the situation may be for family members. Words such as, "Before we get to what's going on with your father, can you let me know how you're holding up in all of this?" can help family members to feel seen and validated.

- Check in often with family members to see if they have questions or concerns about the patient's care.

This is most effectively done standing face to face or sitting with the family, thereby conveying a visible willingness to attune. If it's done in passing or from a distance, it's more likely to be seen as a token gesture rather than representing a sincere wish to be present for the family member.

- Be proactive in the information you share with the patient's family as the team at St. Peter's did with Mary and her family. The staff had reason to assume that Mary might do quite well with just hearing the short version of what was going on with her mother, but they took the time to explain everything to her anyway so that she would feel seen, included, and fully invited to ask questions and express concerns. Because they connected with Mary she rested easier and was able to be there for the rest of her family in ways that would have been compromised if she'd been left to guess about the quality of her mother's care.

Still, holding is far from an exact science, and holding the family is even trickier. As people move through the sometimes terrifying experience of being a loved one's primary support system, they cannot be expected to respond consistently to even the most tried-and-true methods of relationship building.

We are called to respond with authentic curiosity even when our efforts to hold are sometimes rebuffed. In truth, we cannot know what will help a family member feel held, and it's quite possible that in a particularly fearful moment nothing will help. In that moment perhaps we're called to hold as the silent witness, the one who stays present and

It's quite possible that in a particularly fearful moment nothing will help. In that moment we're called to hold as the silent witness, the one who stays present and does not run away.

220

does not run away—even when it seems we are being pushed to do just that.

Years later, Laura still has vivid negative memories of her father's care. She later told us two additional stories, neither of which suggests that her father received terrible care. They are poignant in their subtlety.

What It's Like Not to be Held

At one point during their time in the hospital, a chaplain appeared at the door of her father's room, saying that he had received a call from the nurse to come by to see if he could be of support to them. While the intention was a good one, because there had been neither preparation nor inquiry into whether this was something the family desired, his unexpected appearance at their door brought them more concern than comfort. They politely declined his support, saying they were fine; then they fretted amongst themselves over whether this was a bad sign. Had the nurse sent the chaplain because their father was getting worse?

A second intervention ultimately became rather therapeutic, although not in the way it was intended. A nurse dropped off some pamphlets to educate the family about what to do when a loved one has a stroke. They were told, as the nurse rushed back toward the door, to let her know if they had any questions. When they opened the packet of pamphlets, on the very top was one entitled *Sex after a Stroke*. The patient's wife said wryly to her children, " . . . As if that was front of mind right now!" The entire family collapsed into laughter. The incongruence between their grief and their trying to just hold on and the sudden appearance of the pamphlets in their hands, clearly without thought about what they most needed right now, gave them a belly laugh when they least expected it. In telling the story three years later, Laura said with a twinkle in her eye, "I guess you could say that was therapeutic!"

As you might imagine, the family kept quiet about their fears associated with the visit of the chaplain, and they never bothered to mention the ultimately harmless pamphlet episode. We might be left wondering why they didn't speak up and assert their needs in these instances, especially given how dissatisfied they were with so many elements of their care experience. The answer is fairly simple: they were grieving. They also felt vulnerable and afraid. They'd already had a terrible experience when they'd tried to get a nurse taken off of their father's care. It was reasonable for them to fear that if they offended the hospital staff by speaking up, their father's care might be further compromised.

They were reeling from the events of the past 36 hours, and they were being guided more by emotion than logic. As they experienced the care team turning away from them they turned away themselves, perhaps as a method of self-protection.

In our relationships with family members, it is again beneficial to consciously attend to the concept of a distinct beginning, middle, and end which has been applied throughout this chapter. Family members need the same meeting, greeting, and orientation that patients need, and they need it repeatedly. As care is administered (in the middle phase), explanations of procedures and protocols serve to soothe family members as surely as they do the patient. Family members are often hyper-vigilant on behalf of their loved ones. If we hold them by giving them clear indications about what the patient can expect next, family members often move from red alert to a much lower level of concern.

Seeing Family Members as an Essential Part of the Health Care Team

The care of the patient may be entirely in the hands of his family between clinic appointments and hospital admissions.

If the family system provides physical and emotional support to the individual receiving care, the chance that the patient will follow the care plan and adhere to the medication requirements are improved. In order for the family to provide optimal support they must be included, supported, and educated by the care team.

Collaboration with the patient and family throughout the care experience is an active example of holding. Here are some common practices from the field which, when integrated into care, ensure that family members are included as part of the care team. Notice that the two pillars of all of these essential actions are invitation and education.

- Empower the family as often as possible by continually inviting them into the care processes and educating them about what you're doing on behalf of the patient. When appropriate, teach them how to do the process themselves.

- Provide as much information for the family as is appropriate, anticipating and answering their questions to continually orient them to what's happening with the patient and to seek their guidance when appropriate.

- Let go of seeing the patient's family members—at least those who are core to the patient's recovery and care—as visitors. If the patient has identified a family member (who may or may not be a blood relative) as essential to his recovery, the family member becomes a member of the care team, not a visitor.

Ideally, as you communicate with family members your demeanor conveys a sense of a gathering together of the whole team—a team of which they are a vital part. We say, in effect: "Okay, let's sit down and talk about this together."

Admittedly, responses to our invitations will vary from family to family, and it's even possible that family members who express interest in being included in the patient's care early on may grow weary of the process as it proceeds and become apathetic, resentful, or even hostile. If this happens it's still incumbent upon us to continue to invite family members into the process and educate them as thoroughly as possible about how best to care for the patient. If the response we get is not positive, we know that the family member is in need of our care in that moment. We check in to see what the family member is struggling with, attune ourselves to his or her current state of being, and work on being there for and with the family member. While this may appear to be too time consuming, it may help to remember that proactive engagement will likely save time in the long run, reinforce care that is necessary for the patient's recovery, and perhaps even prevent readmissions.

Overcoming Obstacles to Involving the Family in the Care of the Patient

Skilled clinicians facilitate family involvement in the care of the patient by building on family members' strengths while respecting the differences in their relationships, coping methods, and individual circumstances. We do our best to honor racial, ethnic, cultural, age, and socioeconomic diversity in all families. Some ways to do this include:

- Remain flexible and adaptable, being ready to make special arrangements to include family members in the patient's care if necessary. For example, if the patient's family doesn't speak the language spoken by the clinician, the clinician holds the patient's family by securing interpreters when needed. If the patient's family members require special accommodations because of disabilities or other difficulties, acknowledge and accommodate these needs whenever possible.

- Remain cognizant that you may be challenged by what you may perceive as a lack of caring, shirking of responsibilities, excessive difficulties, or excuse-making by family members. In the face of these behaviors your work is to wonder, follow, and hold these family members. A moment of your undivided attention or nonjudgmental witnessing of their difficulties may be enough to help them pull themselves together enough to care for their ailing loved one.

One of our favorite stories is about a care team going the extra mile to care for a family in the Neonatal ICU unit at a large hospital on the West Coast.

Not a Code Gray

A young woman gave birth to a baby with severe congenital anomalies incompatible with life. The plan was to provide the baby full treatment for ten days. If she continued to deteriorate despite aggressive treatment, treatment would be withdrawn and the baby would be allowed to die. The parents were both gang members and responded with threats and anger when they were told the bad news about their baby's condition and that the aggressive treatments were seen as potentially futile by the medical experts.

In the past, this would have been a case that security, social work, risk management, and hospital administration would have been involved in—likely a Code Gray.

Of course it was "inappropriate" for the family to threaten the care team, but that was hardly the point. Every member of this dying baby's family was suffering, and when the NICU team looked at this large, loud group of intentionally threatening people, they saw an opportunity for profound healing.

Several nurses volunteered to be the primary team for this patient and her family, foregoing some of their scheduled days off to provide continuity of care. The nurses found out that the father was an artist of sorts and they arranged for him to design a scrapbook about his baby's birth and her short, heartbreaking life, and to create artistic items for the parents of the other children in the unit. The nurses knew that the family had few resources, so they pooled their own money to buy the baby a baptismal gown and arranged with the family to have the baby baptized in the unit. All the while this baby was on the most advanced life-saving equipment and received the highest level of technical care available.

By the end of 10 days, the parents and their large family gathered in the hospital. The baby was dressed in the pretty outfit the nurses gave her. She was taken off life support and given to her parents and family to hold in a private area where she died in the arms of her loved ones.

It was clear that the parents were healed from much of their hurt and anger as they took time to hug the staff and thank them for the great care they provided their baby but also for them. The staff was invited to the baby's funeral and two of the primary nurses attended.

All the reverberations from this unit's intervention with this one family will never be fully known, but it doesn't take much imagination to realize that each member of this family felt more loved after this heart-rending event than they had before. What happens to people when they find out that they matter this much to people to whom they long assumed they were invisible?

What happens to people when they find out that they matter this much to people to whom they long assumed they were invisible?

In our work, it is a unique honor to offer the gift of our full attention, our attunement, our sincere wonder, our willingness to follow, and our intentional holding to people who are in dire need of it. In our work with clinicians from around the world we are told again and again that this is the very reason they were drawn to health care in the first place.

Language for Holding

While the intention behind our words is always of paramount importance to how they will be received, intention is perhaps never more important than it is in holding.

Understanding the language of holding can be this simple:

- Language that builds connection helps to create an experience of holding.

- Language that fosters disconnection diminishes holding.

This is language that fosters disconnection (Adapted from Lown, B., 2007, p.36):

Father: Where's my son? What's happening with my son? I've been waiting here for hours and no one has come out to talk to me! What's the matter with you people? There is no excuse for this! Where's my son?

Clinician: Sir, you have to calm down. You're not making things any easier.

Father: I'm not going to calm down. I want to know what's going on with my son!

Clinician: We'll tell you, but I don't appreciate your talking like this. I've been up all night with your son.

Father: I don't care. I've been up all night too!

This conversation is going nowhere. The clinician is addressing a part of the father's brain (an ancient, reptilian core that is designed for action in response to perceived danger) that will be absolutely unresponsive to the clinician's words. At best the father might pick up a shred of stray empathy in the clinician's voice and begin to soothe himself. More likely, father and clinician will not make a connection. The clinician will walk off, sighing about this irrational and unappreciative parent, and the father will storm off or sulk in his waiting room chair, feeling unheard and building up a head of steam for the next clinician who enters his field of vision.

It's not that the clinician is intentionally creating disconnection; it's that in circumstances in which people are frustrated or angry, connection must be intentionally built in order for people to feel seen, heard, and held.

The clinician above doesn't know some very important things about the father. The little boy has a long history of severe asthma with multiple exacerbations and trips to the emergency room, but this is the first time his son has ever required an ICU admission. Watching his son struggle to breathe, and the subsequent intubation procedure, has terrified the father. He has been in and out of the ICU asking questions of anyone he can find. He has been sitting alone in the ICU waiting room for what feels like an eternity.

In circumstances in which people are frustrated or angry, connection must be intentionally built in order for people to feel seen, heard, and held.

As always, however, there's more to the story. This is language that fosters connection (Lown, B, 2007, p. 37):

Father: Where's my son? What's happening with my son? I've been waiting here for hours and no one has come out to talk with me! What's the matter with you people? There is no excuse for this! Where's my son?

Clinician:	Mr. S., I'm Dr. N. (*He reaches out to shake hands, sits down, and signals his intention to listen.*)
Father:	I've spent three hours down in the emergency room and now five hours up here in the ICU. I've asked the nurses and the doctors and they all say, "We'll be right with you." But no one has come out to talk with me all this time. I want to know what's going on with my son!
Clinician:	I'm sorry. I thought somebody had come out to speak with you.
Father:	Well obviously no one has spoken with me. I know nothing. What's going on with my son?
Clinician:	I'll tell you. (*He speaks quietly and slowly, arms resting in his lap.*) We've had the pulmonary specialist come in. He's been working with your son. We've all been working with your son, and he is beginning to respond.
Father:	Well that's certainly a relief. But that's no excuse. This is wrong! I shouldn't have to wait and I'm very angry.
Clinician:	It *is* wrong. You have every right to expect that we would communicate with you about what we're doing, and about your son's condition. It's not right that you have been left to wonder and worry alone.
Father:	His brother had the same thing, you know—two years ago. I waited hours before someone came out and told me he had died.
Clinician:	(*He reaches out to touch Mr. S.'s shoulder.*) Oh, Mr. S., I'm so sorry. (*He waits quietly until Mr. S. is ready to speak.*)

In this revision of the interchange the clinician decides to abandon the quest to make the father change his behavior. He stops taking the father's anger personally. He makes room for the possibility that the anger had meaning in the father's world. He lets his posture and affect take care of the job of soothing the father (something words alone are notoriously ineffective at achieving), while his words respond directly to the father's stated worries.

The clinician follows. As a result, he connects. He entered the father's world instead of demanding that the father obey the rules of the clinician's world.

The immediate result of following in this case is that the father is soothed and feels part of the treatment. The nurses and doctors have more time to devote to direct care.

The longer-term result is that the father is happy with the care at this hospital, is more likely to follow through with aftercare recommendations, and will readily return for care to this place where the people treated him as a person.

There is also one more very long-term result: A clinician experiences the truth about anger—that there is always a reason for anger no matter how unreasonable the feeling appears to be. There is always a back story, and sometimes that back story will knock you right out of your chair if you make a connection and take the time to find out about it.

In the lists that follow, we've included both the language of holding and language that diminishes holding. The language of holding is more complicated and nuanced than that of wondering or following because holding is so necessarily individualized, guided by the person, guided by what we learn and hear through our wondering and following. That said, there are fundamental characteristics of the language of holding:

- It's language that's focused on what is important to the other.

- It's validating language.

- It's language that moves into action and that's based on what the person needs.

Holding is not passive, and neither is the language of holding. The language of holding affirms the individual's experience, focuses on the needs of the other, makes no excuses, and puts up no defense. The language of holding may also include apology. For more on the therapeutic uses of apology, see Appendix D on page 396.

Language that Fosters Holding:

- I remember when you told me ...
- I'm sorry you had to wait; that's not okay.
- I'm here, and I will ...
- You have every right to ...
- Tell me more about ...
- I will see to it that _____ is done for you ...
- I will help you; let's ...
- This must be terribly difficult ...
- Here's what I know about ...
- Let me go with you and ...
- I will follow through until this is resolved.

Language that Diminishes Holding:

- I'm sorry, but I (insert any excuse)
- I have other patients; I can't be everywhere.
- I didn't know because I wasn't here yesterday.
- I was just trying to help.
- I'm doing the best I can for you.
- I wish you'd called me earlier.
- I'm sorry you had to wait; I have a lot to do today.
- [Colleague] was supposed to take care of that for you.
- (to family) If you don't _____ , I'm going to have to ask you to leave.
- That's not my job.

There's one more aspect of the language of holding that we'd like to shine a light on. It's what we call informed reassurance. Informed reassurance is based in fact and action and offers a specific reason for the patient to be reassured. It conveys the competence and confidence of the clinician and it soothes the patient or family member.

The Language of Informed Reassurance:

- I'm going to help you turn on your side; it will help you . . .
- The pain will subside shortly because...
- We learned from your last appointment how to manage your pain better this time.
- I've seen many people recover from . . . because . . .
- Your mother is surpassing all of our expectations . . .
- You are making great progress.

Summary of Key Thoughts

- Holding is an act of devotion. It's a conscious decision to lift up, affirm, and dignify that which the patient or family member has taught us, resulting in intense focus on the patient or family member while treasuring both the information and the person.

- When individuals in our care are at risk of harm, betrayal, disrespect, or even gossip, we come to their defense. We want what is best for them, and we are prepared to make sacrifices to see that they get it.

- Acts of holding include listening to the patient and remembering over time what he has said.

- Holding happens when clinicians who are attuned to the patient and family are devoted to wondering, following, and doing everything it takes to create a safe haven for the patient and family.

- Holding asks us to carry the experience of the patient gently in our hands, keeping confidences as needed and appropriate, defending the patient against those who would disrespect her, lifting up her story as if it were our own.

- Holding means watching over the patient and family as a sentry, assuring their safety and the quality of their care.

- When we see a patient or family as "difficult" it may be because we have dropped them in some way; the solution is for us to build connection and restore holding.

- Sometimes there is nothing to be done other than to provide a sturdy presence—to be the person who stays both physically and emotionally present when the patient feels untouchable, unlovable, or insufferable. Witnessing is an act of healing.

- Patients and their families are at continual risk for feeling disoriented in a clinical setting.

- When we make sure that every interaction we are part of has a clear beginning, middle, and end, we continually re-orient the patient, which helps him to feel secure and held.

- Transitions are often the times of highest vulnerability for patients—the times at which they are at greatest risk for feeling dropped.

- When your words, affect, and actions all say, "I'm here for you," you're holding the patient, and she feels it and becomes more secure within it whether she consciously notices it or not.

- Holding can happen in any moment when we take the time to do what helps our patients to feel held. Remember Jill Bolte Taylor's Dr. Greer who "took the time"; "leaned down"; "touched"; "watched over me"; "understood"; "treated me with respect."

- In emergency situations, in which patients are often terrified, holding can be established very quickly by sustained presence and informed reassurance.

- People who are very angry will often resist holding the most and are most in need of holding.

- Collaboration with the patient and family throughout the care experience is an example of active holding.

- See the patient's family members as people needing our care and support.

- See the patient's family members as essential members of the care team.

- Overcome obstacles to involving the family in the care of the patient by building on their strengths while respecting the difference in their relationships, coping methods, and individual circumstances.

- Visible expressions of connection between and among members of the care team increase the patient's sense of security. When you and your colleagues are obviously working together, the patient feels held.

- Language that builds connection helps to create an experience of holding. The language of holding affirms the individual's experience, focuses on the needs of the other, makes no excuses, and puts up no defense.

Reflection

- Rita Charon writes, "To know what patients endure at the hands of illness and, therefore, to be of clinical help requires that doctors enter the worlds of their patients." What does this mean to you and your practice?

- Describe a colleague who consistently demonstrates respect, acceptance, and compassion for all patients and their families, even those whom others may experience as difficult and/or frustrating. What do you think inspires and sustains his or her commitment to such a high degree of regard and acceptance?

- Reflect on this passage:

  "It's a reality in health care that we are called to bear witness to sometimes repellent physical illnesses and injuries as well as the often hard-to-be-with emotions that our patients may be feeling. Sometimes we can help by doing, but sometimes there is nothing to be done other than to provide a sturdy presence—to be the person who stays both physically and emotionally present when perhaps the patient feels untouchable, unlovable, insufferable."

  What experiences come to mind as you read the above? What helps you to be present and witnessing in the face of suffering? What helps you cope with your own emotions during such times? Does your team come together to support each other through difficult and painful experiences in caring for patients? What helps you cope together?

- If your patients were asked whether the people caring for them appreciated or respected each other, what might they say? What visible demonstrations of teamwork would they describe?

- Reflect on the contrast between Mary's story of her mother's care (page 209) and Laura's story of feeling as though she and her family were abandoned by the care team (page 213). What do you think is important about the patient's family perceiving that the care team understands the meaning and magnitude of the illness or injury of their loved one?

- Reflect on an experience in which extraordinary measures were taken by you or an entire team of caregivers, in order to create a safe haven for a patient and his or her family in a time of crisis.

- Reflect on Tina's and her mother's experience in the ER (page 206). What contributes to such duplication in information gathering? What prevents the team from collaborating and sharing information? What strategies could alter such an inefficient and dismaying (for the patient and family) process?

- Reflect on your practice. When is holding easy for you, and when is it more challenging?

- Reflect on the statement, "Holding requires each patient encounter to have a beginning, middle, and end." What are the ways in which you attend to these three distinct phases? What challenges you most and why?

- Listen to "Her Name Was Ruth," from the *See Me as a Person* CD, with a group of colleagues and reflect together on what it means to you and whether it inspires any changes in your practice.

- According to research done by Planetree, when hospital staff members are asked to list the attributes of the "perfect patient and family," their response is usually "a passive patient with no family"—one who doesn't ask questions, doesn't ring the call bell, has no visible family member or friends to advocate on his or her behalf, and does exactly what he or she is told. How would you and your team describe the perfect patient and family?

- What are some ways that family members have helped you improve care of the patient?

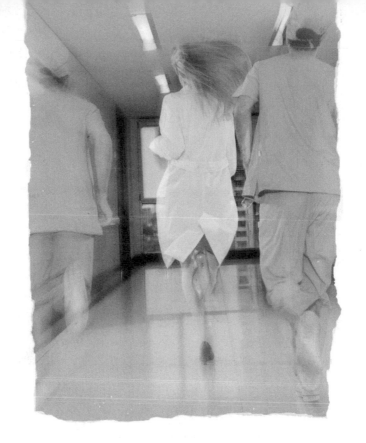

Chapter Six

Moving Beyond Obstacles with Clarity and Purpose

I invite you to sit with this rather radical possibility: Our objectification of patients, their families, each other, and ourselves, is not an effect of the current chaos in health care; it is, in fact, the cause of it.

—GARY SALTUS, CARDIAC SURGEON AND
EXECUTIVE COACH

*T*he interplay of obstacles and solutions is part of the tension of the universe. Light has such status in our lives because we are aware of darkness. We recognize good because we know its opposite. Love stands out as so glorious mostly because we know what hate and apathy look like.

What we have talked about in this book is nearly impossible. It's irrational. We're asking too much. The obstacles against connecting deeply and empathetically with one patient—just this one person in just this one moment—sometimes seem completely insurmountable.

But other times they don't. Sometimes the weather is calm and it's easy to connect. Often, even as the storm rages, you connect anyway. You find your way to your patient or the patient's worried family member and you touch a shoulder, connect eye to eye, and give timely, informed reassurance that instantly helps calm the person and guide him toward healing. You reach across everything that threatens to stand in your way, and you connect.

Still, it is abundantly clear that there are obstacles to providing care that is based on a therapeutic relationship with the patient. Before attending our workshops, participants complete a survey that asks them to identify their greatest challenges to being in a therapeutic relationship with patients and families. They are invited to indicate all that apply from a list of possibilities; they also have the option to write in any additional factors. The challenges listed include personal factors, environmental stressors, and patient-family factors.

Figures 6.1 and 6.2 on the following pages reveal the most significant challenges reported. They represent the responses of more than 300 workshop participants from acute care hospitals across the country over a three-year period. Nurses comprise 85% of the respondents; the remaining 15% are physicians, physical therapists, social workers, pharmacists, respiratory therapists, and occupational therapists.

In response to the question "What personal factors or external stressors challenge your ability or the ability of your colleagues to establish a therapeutic relationship with patients and families?" the two responses chosen most often were time constraints and conflicting priorities (70%) and fast-paced, complicated environments (65%). The third-place response was the clinician's tendency to judge or discount people perceived as demanding and difficult (38%).

FIGURE 6.1: Personal Factors or External Stressors that Challenge the Therapeutic Relationship

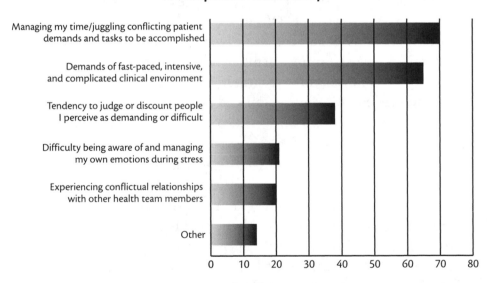

In response to the question "What are the most challenging patient and family interactions for you?" the three most frequent responses all described difficult emotional encounters with the patient and/or family: highly critical or demanding patients and families (88%), families who appear uncaring or potentially harmful to patients (69%), and patients or families projecting anger verbally and/or physically toward the caregiver (61%).

FIGURE 6.2: Patient-Family Interactions that Challenge the Therapeutic Relationship

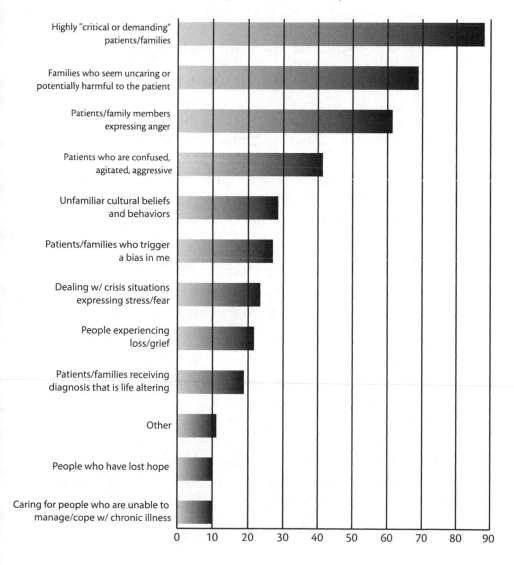

Overall, our surveys consistently identified the same four obstacles regardless of size of the organization, region of the country, or health care discipline. They are:

- **Chaotic Care Environments:** Clinicians define chaotic care environments as fast-paced, intensive, high-stakes environments in which they are consistently burdened by lack of time, limited resources, and competing priorities and tasks.

- **Time Constraints:** Clinicians often identify having difficulty coping with the minimal time allotted for caring interactions within fast-paced health care settings.

- **Patient and Family Anger:** Clinicians find it challenging to remain therapeutic with highly demanding or angry patients and families, including individuals who may seem uncaring or potentially harmful to the patient and/or to the clinical team.

- **The Judging Mind:** Self-reflective clinicians recognize that their own judgments about people and situations can interfere with their ability to remain therapeutic and see the patient and family as people.

In order to put ourselves into a place to therapeutically engage with patients, we believe it is important to explore these obstacles, as well as to reflect on who we intend to be in the face of them. Through such reflection we may increase the possibility that when we encounter the obstacles, we can consciously find ways to think and act which will allow us to stay present and relate therapeutically with our patients regardless of external stressors. As we reflect on the four identified obstacles to therapeutic relationships, we will invite you to look at them through two primary lenses:

- Who am I as an individual in the face of these obstacles? For what am I responsible? For what am I accountable? What is my authority in this situation? What actions can I take? Who and what can I influence? What do I need to release? What is mine to own?

- Who am I as a team member in the face of these obstacles? What can I do to maximize the functioning of my team in a way that supports the most beneficial patient-clinician relationships? What is within my power to influence or change within my team? What is mine to own?

The culture of the organization is a significant factor in creating the best conditions for clinicians to provide therapeutic care. There are clearly best practices in creating such a culture, including those related to the values and beliefs of executive leaders, the mission and vision of the organization, and the practice of keeping a laser focus on humane, compassionate, and clinically excellent patient care (Frampton, Gilpin, & Charmel, 2003; Koloroutis, 2004; Koloroutis, Felgen, Person, and Wessel, 2007; Kovacs, Bellin, & Fauri, 2006). While the organizational domain is outside the scope of this chapter, Appendix E on page 401 offers a summary of successful practices in those organizations that have successfully created the conditions and culture to support the very best patient and family care.

When we feel as though we are drowning in the chaos, in our sense of having no time, in our distress over the anger we encounter, or the wave of conscience we feel when we judge another human being, it becomes difficult to connect human to human with the people in our care. We offer this chapter as a resource for readers to reflect on individually and in teams in order to cope with the challenges you encounter. By engaging in reflection and dialogue, health care teams will gain clarity about what matters most and discover ways to support each other, leading to less chaos, better use of time, and fewer nontherapeutic interactions with patients and families. As individuals, reflection and dialogue help us become more conscious of our own responsibility and power to act. This awareness strengthens our capacity to cope with the stressors in our environment and in our relationships with patients and families without compromising our ability to remain present and therapeutic.

We close this chapter with an exploration of compassion fatigue, a fifth obstacle that is not named as such in our survey because it is the *byproduct* of unrelenting chaos, time pressure, and frustrating and nonproductive encounters with patients and families. It is a byproduct of feeling disconnected from those in our care, from our colleagues, and most importantly from ourselves. We'll look at how to identify compassion fatigue, ways to prevent it, and how to release yourself from it if you find yourself in its grip.

Obstacle One: Chaotic Care Environments

The following excerpt was written by a nurse on one of our surveys inquiring about the daily challenges experienced in providing patient care. This nurse's response represents the frustrations of many in the field encountering what sometimes feels like a mountain of obstacles. Her reality is one we all recognize.

A Mountain of Obstacles

I have way too many tasks and no time to prioritize. I face inadequate or malfunctioning equipment and regular lack of response from support departments. I have too much to delegate and not enough ancillary staff. I am weary of all of the duplicate documentation requirements.

As for leadership? Those in positions of leadership here are unresponsive or absent. The processes and systems don't serve the patients and staff. We are constantly dealing with uncontrolled admissions and transfers. There are frequent, ineffective meetings and demanding, self-centered physicians. I have co-workers who don't carry their share of the work and are consumed with victim thinking. We do not have enough time at the bedside. Automation and technology are both friend and foe.

I experience distractions due to personal concerns and sleep deprivation. I have a sense of the work not being fulfilling and not "what I signed up for." Administration doesn't know my reality and wouldn't care anyway. I deal with difficult and intrusive families. I live with a fear of failure or making serious errors. There is lack of time to attend to patients' emotional needs and lack of time to teach patients and families what they need to know. There is fear and resistance to asking for help.

What happened to your energy as you read this excerpt? How in the world can obstacles such as these be dealt with? How can anyone expect that we would or could make room for human connection when faced with such a mountain of obstacles? In the face of this kind of reality, aren't we doing enough by getting the tasks done and getting people through the system without undue physical harm?

Every day, courageous and determined clinicians answer that question with a resounding "No."

Far more often than not, nothing stops you when you have decided what needs to be done on behalf of the patients in your care. You are the one who moves forward with resolve and clarity of purpose when you encounter things that would overwhelm the average citizen: a patient in the emergency department with a staggeringly complex (and none too pretty) batch of wounds; a family overcome with fear for their loved one, clamoring for answers and reassurance; a critical complication in the middle of surgery; iterations of disease that you have never seen before, but which only inspire you to try something else to meet the challenge. That may be part of what attracted you to health care in the first place. It may be what defines you as a person and as a professional.

Here are some of the things you're telling us about the way you think about your practice:

- "I know who I am; I trust myself; I make my own decisions."

- "Accountability is a personal decision and my professional obligation."

- "I do my best to stay on top of what's happening around me, and I try to manage the unexpected with grace and humor."

- "I've learned that kindness and positive attitudes are contagious and that it only takes one of us to positively 'infect' a whole unit."

- "Every patient, every family member, and every co-worker is important; everyone matters. I have the power to act on that belief."

- "I have learned that I must start by having compassion and respect for myself; then, and only then, can I extend compassion and respect to others."

These comments come from clinicians who were identified by their colleagues as exemplars in therapeutic care—people who seem to find their way through the obstacles. We are intrigued by how such exemplars think because our day-to-day reality is determined to a great extent by how we view the

world and our own power within it. A first step in deconstructing chaos is to take a closer look at what is up to each of
us to own. Once we are clear about
what is ours to own, we can begin
to make intentional choices about
our priorities and actions; we can
also choose to be proactive rather
than reactive.

*A first step in
deconstructing chaos is to
take a closer look at what
is up to each of us to own.*

Transcending Chaos on a Personal Level: What Part is Mine to Own?

The exemplary clinicians' ways of thinking are consistent
with the characteristic of self-differentiation. When people are
highly self-differentiated, they have what psychologists term
an *internal locus of control* (Rotter, 1954). Their sense of what to
do in any given moment comes from inside; it is not based on
what they think others might want them to do.

People with an internal locus of control take ownership
and responsibility for their thoughts, actions, and behaviors.
They are less subject to being "infected" by pressures from
others or to absorb others' stress or anxiety. Their mindset is
characterized by self-empowered thoughts: "I know who I am;
I trust myself; I am responsible for making my own decisions;
I am accountable for the outcomes."

Interestingly, these clinicians, as self-directed as they are,
are extremely comfortable working within interdependent
teams. They don't build silos for themselves. They actively
partner with others and are confident enough to integrate the
suggestions of others and to be unthreatened by different
perspectives. Self-differentiated people are active learners and
understand that they are inexorably connected to the people
they work with and the people they serve. Bowen and Kerr
(1988) speak of the importance of cultivating our capacity for

self-differentiation especially when we are in relationship with others, whether as part of a family or as part of a work group.

> *The higher the level of self-differentiation of people in a family [or group], the more they can cooperate, look out for one another's welfare, and stay in adequate contact during stressful as well as calm periods. (p. 39)*

Conversely, people with an *external locus of control* (those who are less self-differentiated) perceive that others determine how and in what ways they are expected or permitted to act. These people depend on others for approval and acceptance, and if their circumstances are less than ideal they may feel powerless. They often feel controlled, and therefore victimized, by their circumstances. Bowen and Kerr (1988) describe the impact of lower self-differentiation in groups this way:

> *The lower the level of differentiation, the more likely the family [or group], when stressed, will regress to selfish, aggressive and avoidance behaviors; cohesiveness, altruism, and cooperativeness will break down. (p.93)*

Having an understanding of self-differentiation and of the difference between internal and external locus of control will serve us in our own professional development and in the development of our teams. If we're able to look at our individual and team practice through the lens of this understanding, we can improve our ability to move intentionally from thoughts and feelings of victimization to thoughts and feelings of empowerment.

Self-reflection is a key to developing greater self-differentiation. If we pause and reflect on the degree to which we may find ourselves feeling victimized and under the control of others, as compared to feeling empowered and aware of our options in a given circumstance, we will have taken an important step toward mindfully developing self-differentiation.

We invite you to reflect on your own level of self-differentiation by completing this short exercise. Reflect on a current challenging situation in your personal or professional life. When you have a specific situation in mind, ask yourself these questions:

- What part in this situation is mine to own?

- What are the factors that contribute to my feeling empowered or not?

- What is usually going on around me when I'm feeling victimized?

- What thoughts contribute to my feeling victimized?

- What are the internal and external conditions that help me function with a higher level of self-differentiation?

- When I find myself functioning at a low level of self-differentiation, what actions can I take to help me move toward a higher level of self-differentiation (e.g. find a coach or mentor, individual or group reflection, or peer support)?

Higher levels of self-differentiation lead to greater emotional health and personal empowerment. Self-differentiation is not a condition we either achieve or fail to achieve. We all have the capacity for evolving and strengthening our level of self-differentiation, and an important first step is being aware of where we are now. We can then proceed to understand those conditions, both internal and external, that help us move toward a higher state of self-differentiation as well as to understand what happens to set us back.

In the next section, we offer two "ways of seeing" that may help us to shift in any given moment in order to take greater ownership for our thoughts and actions. We'll discuss Marie

Manthey's work on the power of "responsibility acceptance" along with Stephen R. Covey's guidance for a way to enhance our ability to think and act with greater efficacy in any set of circumstances.

Fostering Self-Differentiation through Responsibility Acceptance

Marie Manthey, a respected nurse leader, has made the topic of individual and team empowerment her life's work. In recent years, Manthey has focused specifically on the power of responsibility acceptance in diminishing the experience of feeling victimized by the mounting obstacles in one's life and work. We've adapted the following list of Manthey's ideas for self-reflection and dialogue (personal communication, October 11, 2011). You may wish to work through these individually first and then with your team.

- I know that acceptance of responsibility for my life is both an intellectual and an experiential activity. I cannot simply think myself responsible; I have to actively place myself in the position of being responsible.

- The "closed door of power" (personal or professional) opens only when I actively accept responsibility for myself and my own actions 100% of the time.

- An epiphany occurs when I ask myself the question: "Have I accepted responsibility for my life?" I realize that in those times when I accept responsibility, it is impossible for me to feel victimized. Conversely, in those times when I do not accept responsibility, I feel victimized.

- When I consciously make choices that are grounded in my accepting full responsibility for my own thoughts, feelings, and actions, I find my power expanding, my obstacles diminishing, and my effectiveness growing.

Fostering Self-Differentiation by Envisioning Our Circles of Concern and Influence

The work of author Stephen R. Covey complements Manthey's work by offering another way to understand responsibility acceptance and empowered action. Covey's Circle of Concern and Circle of Influence helps us to be clear about what we can influence and what we can't influence in any given moment (see Figure 6.3 on the following page). This is a vitally important distinction for clinicians who tend to think in terms of "getting it all done" as opposed to realizing that consciously electing not to do something can sometimes result in greater service to the people in our care.

In his book *The Seven Habits of Highly Effective People: Powerful Lessons in Personal Change* (1989), Covey proposes that a pathway to greater self-awareness is to pay attention to where we focus our time, attention, and energy. We can evaluate situations and our ability to be effective based on whether our action will have a direct influence on the situation at hand or whether it is outside of our sphere of influence—something that affects us, but over which we have no control. Covey sums it up this way:

> *Proactive people focus their efforts in the Circle of Influence. They work on the things they can do something about. The nature of their energy is positive, enlarging and magnifying, causing their Circle of Influence to increase.*
>
> *Reactive people, on the other hand, focus their efforts in the Circle of Concern. They focus on the weakness of other people, the problems in the environment, and circumstances over which they have no control. Their focus results in blaming and accusing*

attitudes, reactive language, and increased feelings of victim-
ization. The negative energy generated by that focus, combined
with neglect in areas they could do something about, causes
their Circle of Influence to shrink. (p. 89)

Covey submits that when we focus our efforts on the Circle
of Concern, we give our power away as we expend mental and
emotional energy on things we can't really change. The Circle
of Concern is the worry circle—a place where we spin our
wheels, squander precious energy, and experience a very low
level of self-differentiation. When we move our focus into the
Circle of Influence, we are in a position to take action which
creates a positive forward movement. In this circle we are far
more self-differentiated.

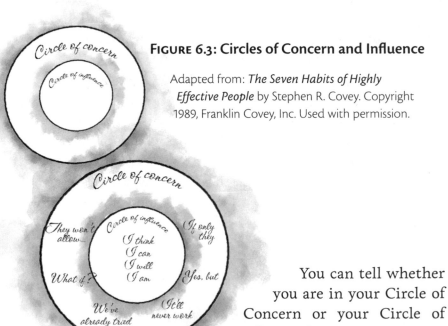

FIGURE 6.3: Circles of Concern and Influence

Adapted from: *The Seven Habits of Highly
Effective People* by Stephen R. Covey. Copyright
1989, Franklin Covey, Inc. Used with permission.

You can tell whether
you are in your Circle of
Concern or your Circle of
Influence by paying attention
to your thoughts and language. If
you are in Concern, your thoughts
and language tend to be other-directed,
negatively charged, and dominated by defeating messages: "if

only they would . . . they always . . . they never . . . it'll never work . . . we've tried it . . . they never listen." If you are in Influence, your thoughts and language tend to be self-directed, action-oriented, positively charged, and dominated by messages of possibility: "I will . . . I think . . . I can . . . we can work together to . . . I will make the time . . . I am here . . . I need . . . I would like you to."

It bears noting that both Manthey's and Covey's work helps us to alter our perceptions of current situations and to focus our attention on what we can do rather than what we can't do. If you find that Manthey's guidance on responsibility acceptance or Covey's Circles of Influence and Concern are helpful tools for you in your work, nothing in your organization can prevent you from applying them. Even if you were the only person on your team to adopt these perspectives, your experience would still improve significantly. Both Manthey and Covey are promoting the possibility that we can intentionally think and act in ways that strengthen our internal locus of control. They offer us principles and tools which we can use to be more self-responsible, self-directed, and empowered.

Transcending Chaos on a Team Level: What Part is Ours to Own?

When clinicians are self-differentiated and focused on that which they can actively influence, they work well within teams. When team members are united around the common purpose of providing the very best in patient care, it becomes obvious to them that teamwork will be necessary to support that shared purpose. It becomes clear that in order to be there for patients and their families, health care clinicians must be there for each other; they must "have each others' backs."

Health care professionals are consistent in their thoughts about working as part of a team. Here is what they tell us:

- "I would rather work short-staffed with a team of people who are all on board than work with a full staff of people who aren't in sync with the reason we're here."

- "When I feel disconnected from those around me, it's up to me to recommit myself to supporting them and thereby restore the connection."

- "My feelings of self-empowerment make me feel more connected to my team."

- "When I am self-directed in my own life and practice, I'm in touch with my calling to be of service to others."

- "I choose to acknowledge that I am inexorably connected, not only to my patients and their families, but to everyone on my team."

We have found that when people hear that they will be working with those whom they consider members of their "A" team—typically defined as people who are positive and helpful, show initiative, are proactive, and are fully engaged—they feel energized enough to take on more, knowing that the time and workload will flow smoothly. If they hear that they're going to have to work with those who demonstrate a victim mentality— defined as those who engage in frequent complaining, show little if any initiative, and demonstrate an apparent apathy toward good patient care or toward helping their fellow team members—they are suddenly "too tired" to take on more, predicting that if they do, the workload will be heavy and the time will be difficult to manage.

A young physical therapist in one of our workshops defined her team as "the best team ever." When we asked her what that meant, this is what she shared:

Characteristics of the Best Team Ever

We never know how the patient will be feeling when he or she arrives for an appointment; we don't know until the patient arrives what happened between the last session and this one. Sometimes we discover that our patient is experiencing some significant problems or distress of some kind and we know we can't rush them through the session without helping them deal with what is on their mind. If we skip past it, it can compromise their session and their longer term recovery.

We know that all we have to do is let one of our colleagues know the situation and the rest of the team will immediately pull together and determine what needs to happen, including covering each other's next appointments if necessary, to assure that we give the patients who presented with unexpected concerns the therapeutic time they need. I call that the best team ever.

We asked how they became such a great team and how they stay such a great team. She said that they've learned who fits on their team and who doesn't. They interview for "fit" which means, in their case, that the individuals must have a strong commitment to compassionate patient care. They deal with conflicts directly so that tensions between team members are not allowed to simmer and get in the way of their practice. She said that addressing conflicts is not easy, but it is worse to work with the tension and dysfunction that unresolved conflicts create. Therefore, they help each other get through it; they consider dealing directly with conflicts a required professional standard. Finally, they take great pride in being the best team ever by doing whatever it takes to provide the very best physical and emotional care possible. She believes this helps to inspire and sustain them, especially when the days get rough.

Self-Assessment: Am I Part of the "A" Team?

This physical therapist described the attributes of an "A" team. We invite you to reflect on your answers to the assessment below and ask yourself this question: Would I be considered a member of the "A" team?

I accept full responsibility and accountability for my practice.	Yes	No	Sometimes
I am reliable—I follow through and do what I say I'll do.	Yes	No	Sometimes
I have a positive mindset, and I take initiative to get things done.	Yes	No	Sometimes
I refrain from nonproductive complaining; if I have a legitimate complaint, I actively seek solutions.	Yes	No	Sometimes
I speak directly and respectfully with anyone with whom I have a problem or conflict.	Yes	No	Sometimes
I do not allow conflicts to interfere with work.	Yes	No	Sometimes
I listen and want to understand other people's perspectives.	Yes	No	Sometimes
I ask for help and I offer help.	Yes	No	Sometimes
I actively participate in team huddles and support my colleagues.	Yes	No	Sometimes
I speak to others with a positive tone and affect, consistently conveying respect and positive regard to all.	Yes	No	Sometimes
I take responsibility for my own learning and development, and I also encourage and support my colleagues' growth.	Yes	No	Sometimes

We invite you to note the pattern of your responses to the self-assessment and reflect on these questions:

- What helps me sustain a high level of contribution to my work and to my team?

- What stops me from making a higher level of contribution to my work and to my team?

- What are some moments or occasions when I have definitely worked as an "A" team member?

- What was it about those times that tapped into the best in me?

- What are some times when I have not worked as an "A" team player?

- What do I need from my supervisor and from my colleagues to help me be an even more valuable member of my team?

- What might I do more of (or less of) to make sure that I am taking care of myself so that I can contribute to my fullest capacity?

Creating a Safe Haven

The following story was told to us by a mother who gave birth to a stillborn son in 2001. This story exemplifies the importance of true teamwork built on a shared purpose and a willingness to go the distance for the healing of the patient and family. The care described in this story took place in a highly complex, highly technical, chaotic and fast-paced tertiary setting. The team "cleared the space" and created a safe haven for loss, grief, and healing to transpire. The team's connection with the patient and family and their connection with each other are what made this exceptional care experience possible.

"They Created a Safe Haven"

The anguish of birthing a stillborn child is beyond comprehension. There is no good way to give such news nor to receive it. Yet we remember our physician's tenderness and compassion as she told us that our son, Micah, would not live. This was the beginning of a heartbreaking journey; nevertheless, we felt seen, safe, and held. The physician said, "I am so sorry. We will get through this together. You don't have to worry about anything. I will take care of all of the details. We have a team of people at the hospital that will support you. You only need to take care of each other and be Micah's parents."

The physician prepared the rest of the team at the hospital by sharing our story with them and paving the way for the care we received to be attuned to our unique needs.

The nurses were present and compassionate in their care, never turning away in the face of our vulnerability, and consistently demonstrating that there was nothing routine about the work they were doing for our family. They supported us and our extended family as well as our community of friends in welcoming Micah into the world, honoring the precious time we had with him in birth and death, and in saying goodbye. We had full permission to do it our way and to know that we were surrounded by people who would take charge and guide us in understanding what was important to us. We could let go and rest into the reality. They created a safe haven.

We were encouraged to spend the hours following Micah's birth holding him, bathing him, baptizing him, talking to him, singing to him. When we decided that it was time to let him go, our nurse came back into the room. Together, along with our family members and a close friend, we offered a prayer of thanks for the miracle and mystery of Micah's brief life.

The safe haven that made all of these caring actions possible was formed through human-to-human connection. The reality of the parents' world and the magnitude of their circumstances were validated by the clinicians' highly connected interactions—not just with the patient and family, but with each other. Because the team was aligned, the parents were held and therefore freed to hold and love their baby during his brief time on earth. They were able to grieve their loss and begin their long journey toward healing.

While highly coordinated, highly attuned teamwork happens when people feel connected, it's important to note that in this case there was also an infrastructure in place to support the team's connection. The team held an interdisciplinary care conference, which they did frequently in situations like this one, to make sure that all stakeholders knew what was going to happen and what would be most therapeutic for this family.

In order to achieve both clinically safe and therapeutically excellent care inside of complex health care organizations, we need each other. This means that it is simply not an option to settle for disconnection, incivility, or lack of collaboration in a health care setting. Positional leaders must articulate clear expectations for all members of the health care team to work with mutual respect on behalf of the patient and to

It is simply not an option to settle for disconnection, incivility, or lack of collaboration in a health care setting.

tolerate nothing less. This is a minimum standard, but to really move beyond the obstacles we have been discussing, we are called to go beyond the minimum requirements. The teams that provide extraordinary therapeutic care, such as the perinatal team who cared for Micah and his family and the physical therapy team who comprise "the best team ever," are devoted to a shared purpose and convey professional respect and regard for all members within their group. They are there for each other in ways that support their individual abilities to be there for the patient and family. They build trust and mutual support. They become a community of caring professionals.

Rallying the Community in an Emergency

M. Scott Peck, in his classic book, *The Different Drum: Community Making and Peace* (1987) proposes that through the building of true community, we can achieve greater self-awareness and a new level of connectedness.

Peck says that times of crisis frequently help individuals to coalesce into a community:

> *Genuine communities . . . frequently develop in response to crisis . . . in the course of a minute a distant earthquake causes buildings to crumble and crush thousands of people to death . . . Suddenly rich and poor alike are working together night and day to rescue the injured and care for the homeless. Meanwhile men and women of all nations open their pocketbooks and their hearts to a people they have never seen, much less met, in a sudden consciousness of our common humanity. (p. 77)*

Peck's observation is confirmed in the stories we hear from health care professionals about those times when their team was at its best. Frequently the stories told are about a code or a flood, the response in New York City to the 9/11 attacks, or a tornado in the town—a time when everyone came forward as a community and teams of people worked side by side, effortlessly and seamlessly. We know what it looks like when we're at our best, but we submit that in these extraordinary instances, it's not just the emergencies or the disasters that bring us together. There is a basic human desire for connection and community within us, and it's this desire for human connection that brings us together. This desire for human connection may lie dormant at times, but it's always there, so it can be awakened whether there is an emergency or not.

What would it take for the amazing teamwork that is described in extraordinary circumstances to become the norm for teamwork during our everyday practice? What would it take for us to come together to meet unexpected emotional needs of our patients and families in the way we respond to codes for unexpected physiological needs? Surely it's not the case that an earthquake victim is more deserving of a united team working seamlessly together than the person who is devastated by her father's massive stroke. What if we came together to support each other when one of us needed to be present with a patient or his family for longer than expected? What if we called "Code Compassion," and everyone in our community of caregivers knew exactly what to do and how to assure that our other patients were not neglected while our colleague focused on the one needing an extra dose of therapeutic attention?

Team Assessment: Gauging Our Team's Level of Connectedness

On the scale that follows, teams are assessed based on their level of connectedness with each other. The three degrees of connectedness are on a continuum from *connected* to *parallel* to *disconnected*.

Connected Team: Members are interdependent and collaborative.			
• Communication is open and direct.	Yes	No	Sometimes
• Relationships are built on trust and respect.	Yes	No	Sometimes
• People are self-responsible.	Yes	No	Sometimes
• Help is offered and accepted as the norm.	Yes	No	Sometimes
• Information is proactively shared.	Yes	No	Sometimes
• Support for each other is consistent and visible.	Yes	No	Sometimes
• Conflicts are resolved and not allowed to get in the way of the work.	Yes	No	Sometimes

Parallel Team: Members are polite but work independently with minimal collaboration.			
• Communication is primarily indirect: through a third party, medical records, or texting.	Yes	No	Sometimes
• People often report feeling "invisible" to other members of the team.	Yes	No	Sometimes
• Help is given when asked for, but rarely offered; therefore people hesitate to ask.	Yes	No	Sometimes
• Information-gathering is duplicated.	Yes	No	Sometimes
• Conflicts are avoided and frequently unresolved.	Yes	No	Sometimes
Disconnected Team: Members are not helpful to each other and relationships are negative and disrespectful.			
• Communication is avoided due to fear and intimidation.	Yes	No	Sometimes
• Power differentials between members of the team are prominent.	Yes	No	Sometimes
• There may be bullying.	Yes	No	Sometimes
• Help is rarely given and done begrudgingly.	Yes	No	Sometimes
• Information-gathering is duplicated and rarely communicated with others.	Yes	No	Sometimes
• Conflicts are unresolved and frequently aggressive and disrespectful.	Yes	No	Sometimes

Where would you rate your team most of the time?

Disconnected Team				Parallel Team			Connected Team		
1	2	3	4	5	6	7	8	9	10

Once you've determined where your team is on this scale, we invite you to reflect on these questions:

- What would your patients and their families say about your team? Would your degree of collaboration and respect for each other be experienced by the patient and family as therapeutic holding?

- What is one thing that you could integrate into your practice immediately that would help you feel more connected to your team members?

- Is it currently within your Circle of Influence to introduce practices to your team that would help build connection? If not, who could you partner with to introduce new practices to your entire team?

- If you scored your team at 7 or higher on this assessment, to what do you attribute your cohesiveness as a team? What will it take to sustain this high level of team functioning?

- If you scored your team at 6 or below on this assessment, what will it take to develop a higher level of team functioning? What can you do? What can you call on your colleagues to do?

In cultures in which teams struggle to work together, fatigue and dispiritedness can easily become the norm. Think back to the idea of an "A" team. The individuals who comprise those highly connected teams actually energize each other and face their challenges together. They experience a collective pride in conquering obstacles and achieving high standards. If you find that you are a member of a parallel or disconnected team and have a vision *Teams are healed one relationship at a time.* for your team to become more connected, the first step is to assess what part is yours to own and what you can personally do in your own relationships to move toward a higher level of collaboration and connection. A second step is to invite others to join you in a shared vision for better team relationships, acknowledging that teams, like individuals, can change and grow. A third step is to realize that teams are healed one relationship at a time; just as negativity is contagious, so are positive energy and healthy interactions. In order to change our reality, we must first see it clearly and honestly acknowledge it. Then we can take clear actions within our own Circle of Influence to live the vision we desire.

Obstacle Two: Time Constraints

We exist in a time-frantic society. Health care cultures are especially driven by time concerns, which are exacerbated by the reality of caring for large numbers of people needing complex interventions, often at the same time, whether it's due to multiple appointments in a clinic setting or the sheer numbers of people assigned to inpatient care teams. Our relationship with time is tenuous, fragile, and even irrational at times. We try to multitask to get everything done. In so doing, however, we may not be present with the person in front of us right now. While it might be true (or so it seems at the moment) that we got more things done in a certain period of time, it is likely that the cost to us is high. Additionally, chances are increased that the people around us will begin to feel invisible or irrelevant. It is also likely that in our distraction and multitasking we increase the possibility of making an error or needing to spend additional time soothing and reconciling with patients or families who felt overlooked.

Entrainment and Time-shifting

Dr. Stephan Rechtschaffen, a pioneer in the wellness movement and the founder of the Omega Institute for Holistic Studies (1996), describes the phenomenon of "entrainment" related to time in the following excerpt from his book, *Time Shifting: Creating More Time to Enjoy Your Life.*

> *Western society has set an overly fast rhythm, a rhythm that varies only in that it is continually getting faster, urging us to do more, produce more, learn more. All our [technology is] geared to the acceleration of an already too-frantic speed. [Our technological devices may be] handy for business and sometimes convenient, but they each add to the speed of the rhythm around us, constantly increasing the pressure—allowing us little time for reflection and none for feelings.*
>
> *This rhythm of fast and still faster is a relatively new phenomenon, and no one seems to know how to vary it. Most of us don't even think of varying it, because society judges it "productive," and because we as individuals are so entrained with it that we don't consciously realize we want to change it. (p. 27)*

The phenomenon of entrainment suggests that we may get pulled into the too-fast rhythm of what is going on around us. Rechtschaffen warns that in health care, our entrainment may cause us to speed up everything we do, simply because everything around us seems to be moving fast. When we are unconscious about this entrainment we become its victim, and so do our patients and their families. If we're moving quickly when it isn't necessary to do so, we may send the message that we're not focused enough to attune to our patients, and they can feel dropped. There are times, of course, when speed is required, and when the speed and efficiency of our action actually helps the patient feel secure. This is not about "fast versus slow"; it's about "conscious versus unconscious."

Once we become aware of the speed at which we're moving, we have the option of exercising choice and "time-shifting" with intention. Rechtschaffen describes using the routine of hand washing between patients as a cue to downshift his rhythm so that he is more attuned to the rhythm of the patient and less entrained to the rhythm of the chaotic external clinical setting. Once we become aware of our relationship with time, we can begin to make choices about proactive actions that will actually save time due to the reduced frenzy of activity and chaotic entrainment.

Once we become aware of the speed at which we're moving, we have the option of exercising choice and "time-shifting" with intention.

In sharp contrast to Rechtschaffen's practice of consciously slowing down to attune to patients, many clinicians report that they have no choice but to entrain to their chaotic work environment because of the expectation that they be always available to respond to their cell phones immediately. In such environments there are no limits of any kind on when clinicians (and therefore their patients) can be disturbed, nor do many feel they can claim the right to mute their phones or otherwise indicate that they should not be interrupted for the next five minutes. It does not seem to matter whether they are involved in admitting a new patient, calming a distressed family, or helping someone cope with a new and devastating diagnosis. The expectation seems to be that they must stop and answer.

We have learned that in some settings this phenomenon is compounded further by the fact that cell phone use by clinicians is entirely unrestricted, allowing for calls and texts from family and friends during patient care time. We heard rationalizations for these practices: "It's a new era and the newer generation of clinicians is accustomed to multitasking in this way" . . . "The use of cellphones for personal business at work is second nature to people these days" . . . "It doesn't really compromise patient care, since everybody multi-tasks" . . . "Patients are used to it."

We find none of these rationalizations compelling since none of them addresses the two core issues: 1) Professionals create boundaries between their personal and professional lives. 2) Cell phones are an interruption to the therapeutic relationship—period.

The research of Ophir, Nass, and Wagner at Stanford University (2009) is quite clear: media multitaskers pay a significant mental price. The researchers put high and low multitaskers through a series of tests and found that the high multitaskers were "suckers for irrelevancy" (as reported in Gorlick, 2009). In other words, the high multitaskers were not able to efficiently screen and sort highly relevant information from information that was defined as not relevant. The researchers found that "people who are regularly bombarded with several streams of electronic information do not pay attention, control their memory, or switch from one job to another as well as those who prefer to complete one task at a time" (Gorlick, 2009, para. 1).

We propose that it is imperative for health care teams to address electronic interruptions in patient care and to find strategies that balance the need for quick access with the need for focus and presence.

This story, from the daughter of an elderly patient, offers a poignant contrast between a patient admission in which clinicians take the time and are focused on the patient and an admission in which clinicians are distracted by multitasking and don't take the time to see the patient as a person. This daughter, observing two separate admissions of her mother in a large tertiary center, was struck by the huge difference in the amount of time clinicians were willing to spend with her mother between Admission A and Admission B.

Admission A

My mother was being admitted to the oncology unit for her second round of chemotherapy. She had been diagnosed with non-Hodgkins lymphoma rather late in the course of the disease and by the time her diagnosis was determined, she was quite frail both physically and emotionally. In her first round of chemo she experienced severe nausea and vomiting and it took some hours to get it under control. So with this second admission she was nervous and very fearful of the chemo.

As we exited the elevator and began walking down the hallway, a nurse standing by the station saw us coming and immediately headed our way. She greeted us, "Hello, I'm Teresa and you must be Elda. I'm your nurse and I'll be administering your chemotherapy," she said as she walked with us to my mother's room. "Mary J., your primary nurse, told me all about you. She is on vacation and will be disappointed that she wasn't here to take care of you. She told me a lot about you—including that you always wear great hats!" My mother smiled and touched the sunflower hat covering her bald head.

Teresa walked and talked slowly. Even as others on the unit sped by, she stayed focused on my mother and walked calmly along with her.

Teresa continued as she and my mother ambled down the hall towards her room, "I know last time was really tough, but now we know exactly what dosage works to stop your nausea and we will start it right away. This time will be different; I predict you will breeze through it." As they entered my mother's room, Teresa said, "Elda, I feel so good about being able to get this quiet corner room for you; you'll have a more restful time and I love how the sun comes through like this. I hope it'll brighten everything." My mom nodded and turned to me (I had another appointment to go to). She said, "You can go on now; I have my new best friend." She and Teresa continued talking and I left the room.

The period of time this all took: about four minutes. It involved one clinician. Mom's IV was started within the next few minutes and her chemotherapy was initiated.

Admission B

My mother was being admitted to the telemetry unit with congestive heart failure secondary to the cancer treatment. She was sent from the doctor's office to the hospital, and I was by her side. We exited the elevator and began walking down hallways bustling with activity. We quietly found our way. We stopped at the nurses' station; a rather stressed unit secretary finally looked up and asked who we were. She then pointed us to my mother's room a few doors from the nurses' station.

When we got to the room we began trying to find our way around—a closet to hang her coat, lights, gown and so forth—when a young nurse literally ran into the room. "Oh," he said, "you're here already. I knew you were coming but thought it would be a while yet; we're very busy today." He barely finished his sentence when his cell phone went off and he ran out of the room saying he would return shortly. I helped my mother get settled into bed and the nurse returned shortly thereafter. As he came into the room, he told her he needed to complete her admission paperwork. He appeared to review the admission form for a few seconds and then placed it on the bedside stand and turned and checked my mother's pedal pulse. At that moment his cell went off again and he exited. My mother looked at me and said, "He is full of himself."

I needed to leave for another appointment and was barely gone 15 minutes when I heard an overhead page asking me to return to the unit. I found my mother sobbing and saying, "I want out of here." It seems that when she asked her nurse when she could get something to eat or drink he responded that she could not eat or drink until after her procedure (a transesophageal echocardiogram). My mother had not even been informed that this procedure was being scheduled or why. Because my mother was distraught and refusing the procedure, her doctor came to the unit and spent 45 minutes explaining the procedure and trying to calm her, but she would not agree to the procedure. Further, she wanted to be transferred off the unit as her trust was shattered. She was transferred to the oncology unit with remote telemetry.

Time for admission B was nearly four hours. It involved four clinicians, plus administrative people.

In Admission A, the admitting nurse was well-informed about Elda and therefore was proactive in meeting her and establishing trust. She was not entrained to the busyness of the unit. The brief time she took was well spent, as not only did it expedite the process, but it put Elda into a more favorable position to tolerate the chemotherapy and to cope with the experience. Admission B was not proactive. The admitting nurse was entrained to the chaotic rhythm of his environment; it seemed not to occur to him that he had a choice to slow himself down to match the patient. The message conveyed to the patient was that Elda's admission to the unit added to the already busy work load. Elda, therefore, became more fearful and felt isolated and unsafe. Finally, when an invasive procedure was casually introduced as the reason she wouldn't be permitted to eat (rather than in the context of a person-to-person interaction to help her to be consciously prepared for it), her trust was lost and could not be recovered.

Events that might reasonably be seen as small and routine to clinicians are almost always huge events in patients' lives. When clinicians rush or are merely perceived by patients to be rushing, patients feel unsafe. After all, if a clinician rushes into a room, it's obvious that she could rush out just as quickly. It seems almost too elementary to say, but simply slowing down physically to a rhythm more attuned with the rhythm and needs of the patient is essential to quality patient care. When we invest time with patients in a proactive way, keeping them informed, demonstrating to them that they are important to us, patients and their families feel held. When patients and families feel held, their needs diminish and time is saved.

Still, we frequently hear that engaging in a therapeutic connection takes too much time and may even be seen as an impossible goal:

- "Many of my days are very challenging as I try to meet the needs of all of my patients. Many times, several situations arise at the same time, and I find it very hard to meet the needs of all in a timely manner. I feel so stressed out and end up feeling like I disappointed my patients and their families, and then I feel incompetent, which really makes me feel bad about myself."

- "With the increase in patient acuity in the acute care setting, it becomes challenging to find time to establish these relationships; patient's clinical needs take priority over emotional needs."

- "There is often not enough time to spend with one patient, to talk or just be with them, because there are so many others waiting for my attention."

In these words you can see the strain of clinicians wanting to do as much as possible within hurried circumstances. The frustration can be high when we feel like we're running behind. However, a quick reflection on Covey's Circle of Influence/Circle of Concern model can help us access a more peaceful rhythm in our work. The comments above suggest that clinicians may be putting too much of their attention on their Circle of Concern—focusing on "everything there is to do" instead of how they can make the biggest positive difference for each patient in each moment. Conversely, if these clinicians could keep focused within their Circle of Influence—on the things that they can actually change or control—it will help them to prioritize more effectively. Most importantly, it will help them make a choice to let go of those things that are not practical to do. The clinician who feels discouraged and guilty about himself is likely to be stressed over what he hasn't done. The truth is that not every action serves the patient's healing; prioritization helps us learn how to let go of nonessential activities.

Not every action serves the patient's healing; prioritization helps us learn how to let go of nonessential activities.

The following voices from the field are from clinicians who completed a survey asking about ways they dealt with the challenge of time constraints. These clinicians were from a pool of people identified by colleagues as exemplars in patient care. Notice how they make choices about what they will do. Each demonstrates a focus that stays solidly within the Circle of Influence.

- "My main strategy is not overly complicated: I stop and think and ask myself what is the most important thing I need to do at this moment? Is it something that involves safety for a patient, a question that needs to be answered, or do I need to sit with someone having a hard time? I triage and prioritize."

- "Being flexible is key. I set my schedule in the morning and try to follow it, but if something changes I look for an alternative path that meets patient goals. I try to flex my schedule for other colleagues who may need help on a certain day so that if I need help I feel free to ask them, but actually I find people will offer me help, especially if I have helped them in the past."

- "I try to assess who needs the most time, when they need it, and how to prioritize the time. I also remember that every encounter can be therapeutic even if it is short, interrupted, or un-scheduled. If I see the person in front of me right now and am present, it makes a big difference. I have experienced that five minutes seated at the bedside with each patient to plan care for the shift makes a big difference in the way time is spent for the rest of the shift. These five minutes help with the development of the therapeutic relationship, as the patient and family seem to appreciate that I make that time a priority and give them my undivided attention for those few minutes."

- "I always speak face-to-face, with good eye contact, to my patients and families. I tell them what I hope to accomplish, step by step. I must get their buy-in. I am always aware of the needs of the family as well as the patient. This connection makes care go more smoothly. In fact, I find that partnering with the patient's family prevents interruptions and results in a smoother course. It seems as though they are calmer and more invested in the plan."

- "Although some people think caring takes 'too much time,' I have experienced that the opposite is true. Focusing on the patients' priorities and what matters to them will help them participate more actively in their healing process. Therefore, even though more actual time may be taken initially, I noticed that, eventually, more time is saved in caring for patients. I didn't believe this was possible before I experienced it for myself."

- "I begin most interactions with patients by saying, 'What is on your mind right now?' I sit and connect. I am conscious about being present. I find that by giving the person such focused attention, I am able to efficiently assess what is most important to the individual and to involve them in determining the priorities for the day. Consciously connecting person to person saves time in the long run."

In each of these statements, the clinician is focused on what can be done, rather than on what will be left undone; each is working within his or her Circle of Influence. These clinicians and others like them have demonstrated time and again that it's a myth that relationships can't be built with patients and their families because of time constraints. Caring happens in a moment. Each of us has experienced very brief encounters that have stayed with us for a lifetime. The clear message from the exemplars is that an initial investment of time results in greater efficiency in the long run.

Five Minutes at the Bedside—One Small Investment in Human Connection that Yields More Time than it Takes

"Take the time it takes so it takes less time."

—PAT PARELLI, HORSE TRAINER

We teach the importance of taking approximately five minutes seated at eye level with each patient, connecting with what is important to this specific person, partnering with him on the best plan for the day or until you are with him next. The five-minutes concept aligns with Brafman and Brafman's research on instant connection (2010), which emphasizes that proximity, resonance (which we've been calling attunement), and safety are all accelerators of connection. Additionally, research from the University of Kansas Hospital (2010) linked physicians sitting at the bedside with increased patient satis-faction. Patients perceived that physicians spent more time with them and were more interested in them when the physi-cians sat down. This was reported even when the physicians' actual time seated in the room was less than the time they spent in the room standing.

One of the most effective and simple proactive strategies is partnering with the patient and family by meeting with them and agreeing on what is most important for the time you are with them. Everyone knows that unexpected things will happen that can disrupt the best-laid plans, but when a patient's top priority is identified, she can be sure that at the very least, the one thing she identified during the meeting as *most* impor-tant will be taken care of. This helps patients feel seen, held, and well cared for, and it can also help clinicians experience a greater sense of accomplishment in their practice.

This is something that clinicians can practice no matter what culture they're in. It's a one-to-one "contract" that takes five minutes of attunement (undivided attention) and a will-ingness to wonder (by inquiring), follow (by listening and acknowledging), and hold (by delivering the one thing that is most important to this individual patient). The plan may be carried out by the clinician herself, or aspects of it may be delegated to other members of the team. The key is that the primary clinician follows up and makes sure the need was met and the commitment fulfilled.

When we discuss five minutes at the bedside, a common question arises: What about overly talkative patients and families?

Those who have had this experience know the feeling of being trapped and unable to stop the flow of words and the many needs and worries that some patients and family members express. Fortunately, there is an effective way to set limits with those individuals who are particularly verbal and pose a challenge to your ability to attend to all of your other patients. If the person is simply not aware that he is overly talkative and therefore does not limit himself or is not comforted by the attention given, the clinician must take the lead and set boundaries. This is done by proactively stating the time parameters and signaling through firm language or touch when the time is up. "Mr. S., I want to listen to what you're telling me. I must move on to my next patient. I will be back at ____, and we'll continue then." It is important to return when you say you will. When given your structured, focused time, the people who "don't stop talking" may be more willing to listen to and respect practical limits, as they no longer feel they have to fight to be heard.

When there are patients (and sometimes family members) who experience emotional distress, they may require an extended amount of time from a clinician (to air concerns, to deal with grief or fear related to a new diagnosis, or to deal with any of the many normal and unique human responses to stress and illness). This is frequently unplanned or unexpected time. As was a norm for the "best team ever" described by the physical therapist earlier, it makes sense for all health care teams to have a mechanism in place to back each other up so that when one clinician needs to spend extended time with a person experiencing fear, anxiety, or difficulty coping, he knows that his other responsibilities are not being neglected.

Consider what it would take to create a "Code Compassion" within your care team. Like the codes called for physiological distress, a Code Compassion would be a signal to your team that a patient needs emotional support to cope with her illness or acute crisis. What would it take for such a signal to be conveyed and for the entire team to understand what it means: that the team makes certain that all patients continue to receive supportive and safe care while the clinician who called the Code is allowed to be fully present with the person needing emotional support? The clinician could be fully present because she would know that none of her other patients will suffer, because her colleagues have her patients in their care.

As with chaos, it may be that the most important way to deal with the obstacle of time constraints is by reflecting on our own relationship with time in order to see that relationship more clearly. It's quite possible that many of us see ourselves, at least occasionally, as time's victim. In those moments we're not seeing our relationship with time accurately. Once we accept responsibility and commit to seeing our situations differently we can see that there are in fact many things we can do in order to work with time more proactively. It may start with the simple exercise of envisioning a work day that flows easily. Ask yourself these questions:

- What would it look like for me to walk through my work day calmly and mindfully by pausing occasionally and tuning into my breath?

- What is one simple thing that I could do to feel less rushed?

- Who on my team could I partner with in my reflection on this issue? Who either shares my dilemma or seems to have mastered it?

Many of the insights we have shared about dealing with chaotic environments can also be useful to those dealing with time constraints. For example, clinicians who are working within their Circle of Influence, and are therefore less drained by a fruitless expenditure of energy within their Circle of Concern, will likely feel less battered by time constraints. Similarly, those who accept responsibility for their own thoughts and actions have a greater chance of being proactive with their time. These are the clinicians who are most likely to engage in time-saving, relationship-building practices such as five minutes at the bedside.

Obstacle Three: Patient and Family Anger

The stories we hear about angry, disruptive patients and families are almost as prevalent as the stories we hear about the chaotic environments in which we are expected to remain focused on patients' sometimes inexplicable demands. It's likely that in your own practice you've had many moments in which you were able to suspend your judgments and connect person to person with people in these situations. It's also likely that there are times when your buttons get pushed and it's all you can do to retain your professionalism.

There is consensus among health care professionals that they are encountering more anger and frustration among patients and families in recent years. It seems to be related to the high volume and task-based focus of many health care settings in which people feel overlooked and clinical staff are vulnerable to feeling overextended, overwhelmed, and under-valued. Concomitants of patient anger, according to the literature, include high expectations of nursing presence and availability, lack of attention to patients' physical and/or psychological needs, and failure of health care professionals to recognize the uniqueness and wholeness of individuals (Plaas, 2002; Shattell & Hogan, 2005).

Literature on anger and illness correlates the root cause of anger with fear and vulnerability (Smith & Hart, 1994; Thomas, 2003). Groves (1978), in a classic article entitled "Taking Care of the Hateful Patient," says that clinicians must understand that underneath the angry demands are deep fears of abandon-ment. That understanding—one that is widely accepted but often forgotten in the heat of the moment—offers us a guiding principle for prevention and intervention that is grounded in our ability to anticipate and recognize anger as fear. With this perspective guiding us, we can respond by connecting rather than giving in to our more automatic response of disconnecting through withdrawal (flight) or confrontation (fight).

Expressions of anger experienced in the health care setting range from mild distress to rage and aggression. The etiology of anger ranges from the normal human response to illness—fear and vulnerability—to pathological origins such as mental illness, addiction, and cognitive changes.

The story below from a nurse in one of our workshops, while not an everyday occurrence, is one you may relate to.

The Meanest Patient in the World

We had had it with this man. He was without a doubt the meanest patient in the world! None of the nurses wanted to care for him. He cursed at us, threw things; he even tried to hit us. It was ridiculous.

Dr. H., a surgeon, overheard us talking about the patient. He wasn't Dr. H.'s patient, but Dr. H. was really interested and asked us to tell him what was going on. After he listened to us, he quietly walked down the hall and into the man's room.

We (the nurses) kept walking past the open door to make sure Dr. H. was OK. Dr. H. was sitting by the man's bed watching television. He sat there for a while, and finally the man said, "What in the hell are you doing in my room?" Dr. H. replied, "Watching television with you." The man said, "Why? Do you like that program?" Dr. H. shrugged, "Not particularly." They were quiet. Then the man said, "I hate it here." Dr. H. looked at him and asked, "Why do you hate it here?" The man replied quietly, "People die here."

We don't know what else was said after that. But we do know that after his conversation with Dr. H., the man was no longer the meanest patient in the world. He was peaceful and cooperative.

I learned that day to love the "mean patients," because I understood that the meanness was fear in disguise. Now I'm the one who volunteers to care for the "difficult" ones. I'm interested,

I'm curious, I know what fear looks like, and I know what to do with it even when it happens to show up as anger and hostility.

The fears and discomforts of a person's life are sometimes suspended in times of crisis; but more often than not, they're multiplied.

The fears and discomforts of a person's life are sometimes suspended in times of crisis; but more often than not, they're multiplied. The caregiver doesn't deserve to be met with anger, but the caregiver *is* often met with anger, and we need to be knowledgeable about the etiology of anger in order to respond to it therapeutically.

Recognizing Anger as a Potent Projection of Fear and Powerlessness

Over the past two decades, Mary has asked health care professionals in her workshops to share stories of meaningful interactions they've had with patients and families. Based on these stories, she's also asked them to attempt to identify the underlying human responses to illness or crisis embedded within the stories. Over time, what came to the surface was that it did not seem to matter what the specialty or diagnosis was; it was clear that there was a "top five" list of human responses to illness and/or crisis that were consistently identified across the spectrum:

1. Fear

2. Grief and loss

3. Pain (physical, emotional, and spiritual)

4. Difficulty coping

5. Powerlessness

Anger is a symptom common to all of these normal human responses to illness—anger in response to fear; anger as part of grief and loss (loss of self, of function, of life as it once was, of a loved one); anger in response to pain which is unrelenting and/or not managed well; anger in response to feeling out of one's comfort zone, unable to cope with the limitations, the pain, the life changes; and of course, anger in response to feeling powerless and out of control. Spiritual author Marianne Williamson (1994) writes poetically about the relationship between anger and fear:

> Anger is one of fear's most potent faces. And it does exactly what the fearful ego wants it to do; it keeps us from receiving love at exactly the moment when we need it most. Our greatest need, when fearful, is to be able to express how scared we are. Instead, of course, we are often tempted to express anger, meekly hoping that somehow, someone will read our minds and say, "I know you're only angry because you feel so scared. Come here and I'll love you." There are those rare moments when the other person is evolved enough to do that; in the vast majority of cases, however, our anger will send others further and further away from us, increasing our pain and increasing our terror. (pp. 134-135)

The fear of illness, like the fear of death, is deep and primal, yet it is never far from the surface. It manifests in expressions of overt anger or expressions of covert anger such as withdrawal and depression. Rita Charon (2004) asserts that effective care of a patient depends on the clinician's capacity to understand and be informed by the human experience of fear. She describes a patient who expressed her fear through withdrawal and depression. Dr. Charon connected with Mrs. M. by focusing on the strength she demonstrated by simply getting up every day and facing the world and her illness by keeping appointments. Charon writes about the importance of staying connected to a chronically ill and depressed patient, despite how uncomfortable it can be:

> ... *Our conversation about the blood tests, electrocardio-graphs and pills was much more brisk and efficient by virtue of our having started with her life and her mood and her fears. In effect, our medical business, by being informed by her over-whelming fears about illness and death, could proceed more effectively because I now knew how desperately she feared illness ... More important in developing an effective thera-peutic alliance than any technical skill was, I believe, my ability to tolerate Mrs. M.'s profound depression and not to flee from it because, of course, to flee from her feelings is to flee from her. (2004, p. 26)*

We've used an example here of extreme depression (anger turned inward), and we've already talked about how difficult it can be to stay present and attuned to people in distress who are experiencing strong emotions of any variety. When people are depressed and withdrawn, it's likely that they will not appear to be inviting us into their world. Now put yourself in Char-on's shoes and ask yourself this question: If Mrs. M.'s symptom of fear had presented as overt anger and resistance rather than withdrawal and depression, would it be easier or more difficult for you to stay present with her?

It's not much of a stretch to see that overt depression is a symptom of fear, grief, loss, pain, difficulty coping, and power-lessness. But what would happen if we thought of overt anger as an emotional symptom of fear, grief, loss, pain, difficulty coping, and powerlessness? What if instead of personalizing it or becoming fearful ourselves, we were able to wonder about what it means, about what is being conveyed by the anger? What if we saw anger as an emotional equivalent to

What if we saw anger as an emotional equivalent to bleeding?

284

bleeding? We don't react to, judge, or disconnect from the person who begins to hemorrhage; we move into right action in response to the symptom of bleeding. We see it as physiological distress, and we don't order the bleeding patient to "stop it and calm down" as a condition of our being kind or of our providing needed services. We see bleeding (just about as messy as anger, when you think about it) as a symptom—not an assault on us or an affront to us.

While we are deep in wonder about another person's expression of anger, we cannot be adversely affected by the anger of the person. Dr. H. did not see the "meanest patient in the world" as someone who was out to make his life more difficult. He saw the man's anger as a symptom of emotional distress, and like Dr. Charon, he did not flee from this person's feelings. Instead he moved toward the person in front of him. What he uncovered was fear, and by being able to name his fear, the "mean" patient was able to release it. As his fear diminished, so did his meanness and anger.

It bears noting that none of this could have happened unless Dr. H. had been curious—not so much about anger (or meanness), but about the person expressing that anger. Dr. H.'s decision to be with the person changed everything, but there were no guarantees that it would. It was always possible that Dr. H.'s presence would not have resulted in such amazing resolution for the patient. It was possible that nothing would change, and Dr. H. knew it. His capacity to move toward the "mean patient" was likely grounded in his understanding of fear and in his ability to not be attached to a specific outcome. He was willing to wonder. Releasing the need to fix this patient, whom the nurses had deemed beyond hope, meant that Dr. H. could be in relationship with the man with openness and acceptance, without any investment in the results. Since his sole aim was to listen and learn, it was unlikely that he would fail.

Factors that May Trigger Patient and Family Anger

Based on our conversations and experiences with people receiving health care, as well as people providing it, we have identified some patterns that exacerbate fear and powerlessness and engender anger in patients and their family members. We believe it is important to consider those factors that we know may trigger anger so that, when possible, we can take action to prevent it rather than unwittingly or unconsciously inciting it. We have organized these patterns into four general categories and illustrated them in Figure 6.4 below.

1. The patient's and family's established patterns of emotional response

2. The patient's and family's back story

3. The patient's and family's previous experience of safety and care in health care settings

4. Points of vulnerability for the patient and family during an episode of care

FIGURE 6.4: Anger and Illness

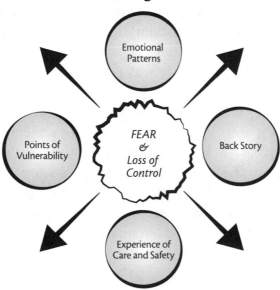

As you can see, the first three factors are about "what the patient comes in with," and the last item is about what happens during the most potentially frightening moments in the patient's care. Clearly we have no control over the patient's patterns of emotional response, back story, or previous experiences in a health care setting. However, our awareness that the majority of what may trigger patient and family anger is related to their previous experiences is an excellent reason to be curious about who they are as people and to follow closely as they offer clues about their unique considerations and concerns. As you read about the four factors that trigger patient and family anger, we invite you to reflect on how often you wonder about these factors on behalf of your patients and their families.

The Patient's and Families' Patterns of Emotional Response

We meet people exactly where they are in their life journey, and they come to the care experience with a long history of emotional responses. Their history is grounded in their experience with being loved and cared for (or not). Patterns are formed based on the ways in which their experiences in their family system cultivated trust or mistrust, attachment or abandonment, acceptance or rejection. Has the family of origin cultivated a core sense of worthiness or a lack of self-worth? Do they believe they are worthy of receiving loving care?

When we are suddenly dependent on others for our care, emotional patterns of response originating in our own family systems will surface and will affect the way we respond to caregivers. This is exhibited in the following frustrating encounter with a patient as described by one of our workshop participants:

Nothing I Said Got Through to Him

This man put his light on and I responded from the nurses' station. He was clearly upset and charging that we were being unresponsive, so I immediately put the phone down and went to his bedside.

You can imagine my surprise when he was angry at me for "hanging up on him!" I hung up the phone to go to him and I kept trying to make him understand that, and we kept going in circles. I said, "I didn't hang up on you. I put the phone down so I could *come* to you."

He replied, "Everybody keeps hanging up on me and no one comes when they say they will. I could be dying here and no one would care!"

I responded, "But sir, I didn't hang up on you; I put the phone down so I could *come* to you." We never broke through the cycle. What can I do with someone like that? I don't think I could have said anything to make him happy!

We explored this interaction with the workshop participants. What was going on here? What would contribute to a grown man being so unsettled by the nurse hanging up the phone? What would break this cycle? The answer, when we stop trying to defend ourselves or convince the man of anything at all, is simple: we listen. In his own way, he is being awfully articulate. His message (and perhaps his long-standing pattern of emotional response) is clear: "I feel abandoned. I can't be sure I know where my lifeline is. Who will save me if I get into desperate straits? Who will hear my call?"

Suddenly we find our words changing. Suddenly we remember the healing power of following: "Oh, my goodness, you thought I hung up on you. You thought I had left you all alone. You had no way to know that you had done it just right—to call me in the way you did—and that I was on my way to help you. You must have been very frustrated after you heard that 'click.'"

Patterns of emotional response cannot be counted on to follow the rules of reason and logic. Because our patterns of emotional response were formed long ago, many of them were formed while we were too young to be rational, and as we suggested earlier, it's not uncommon for patients to regress when they're in deep distress. In the story the nurse told, she was trying to apply reason and logic in a situation in which reason and logic were not something the man could even understand right then, much less appreciate. The language of following allows us to get through to our patients in ways that sometimes nothing else can; for one thing, the language of following is never used to tell anyone he's wrong.

Patterns of emotional response cannot be counted on to follow the rules of reason and logic.

The Patient's and Family's Back Story

We may or may not learn specifics about any one person's back story in a fast-paced care setting. However, it is vital to remember that everyone has a back story and that the person's individual back story is affecting his or her emotional response.

Sometimes we don't need to know the back story. Sometimes it's enough to imagine it. Recall again the man's fear (masked as indignation) at being hung up on. Is it difficult to imagine that he had been in that position before? Can we picture him as a little boy who reached out once when he was particularly vulnerable and terrified and no one was there? Can we imagine that old feelings of powerlessness and aloneness have been awakened on this day in that hospital bed?

Do you remember the story in Chapter Four (page 143) about the patient's sister who was being so "demanding"? When the nurse stopped and listened to her she learned that the sister had promised her mother that she would watch over her little sister. What was seen as demanding and picky by the staff was actually the sister fulfilling an important promise. When you know her back story, you may actually see that her constant complaining is an act of personal integrity on her part. Like the "meanest patient," once the sister was invited by the nurse to put voice to her fears, her anxiety subsided and her actions changed. She felt seen as a person, understood, and supported. She could let go of her brittle vigilance and let the care team help her.

By wondering about the back story (whether we discover it or not), we become more able to attune, follow, and hold the other with compassion, which facilitates the release of anger and opens up the possibility of trust, connection, and ultimately, healing.

Previous Experience of Safety and Care in Health Care Settings

You can imagine that if your loved one did not receive humane and compassionate care in a previous hospitalization, you may be on alert to assure that this time will be different.

It would be irrational to decide that all hospitals are uncaring or unresponsive because the last one—the one that treated your loved one as if she were a nuisance—was. But it doesn't matter at all that it's irrational. That's how we human beings think, especially when the issue at hand is so emotionally laden. The patient's family members may come across as aggressive and antagonistic when what they mean to say is, "Is my loved one safe with you? Do I dare put my loved one into your hands? What if terrible things happen again, like they did in that other place?"

A workshop participant told us about an anesthesiologist who seemed to understand acutely the importance of previous health care experiences on the current experience. He would sit at eye level with his patients and appeared to have all the time in the world for them. He conveyed genuine interest in how the person was doing and asked her to talk about whatever was on her mind: any questions she may have about the surgery, but also any concerns that may be affecting her right now. He brought his authentic wonder to these relationships, asking, "What, if anything, was difficult for you in your past surgeries? I want to understand what it was like for you so I can do everything possible to make sure this time is not difficult for you." This physician recognized the impact of past experiences on the current surgical experience, and by bringing anything that was problematic into the light, he could partner with the patient and take action that would dissipate any anxiety and fear that may compromise the current surgical experience. (Would we be surprised to learn that this anesthesiologist was also known for his singing to patients in the operating room as they were being prepared for surgery?)

Points of High Vulnerability for the Patient and Family during Care

There are predictable points in a care experience that potentially increase anxiety or heighten a person's feelings of fear and powerlessness:

- Admission to the hospital

- Persistent emotional or physical pain

- Immobility

- Dependence

- Surgery

- An invasive procedure

- A new diagnosis

- Enduring many tests without obtaining a diagnosis

- A first appointment

- Transition from an acute care setting to a long term care facility

- A difficult therapy session

- A call or visit from a financial counselor to discuss payment and insurance

- Countless other such moments of meeting, transitioning, and coping

Understanding and remembering these points of vulnerability makes us able to be more consciously attuned during these times and, therefore, more proactive. What is striking about these points of vulnerability is that in the eyes of the clinician they are routine parts of a work day; however, for the people receiving care they are anything but routine and may in fact be life-changing moments.

Shirley MacLaine, playing Aurora Greenway, the distraught mother of a dying daughter in the 1983 film *Terms of Endearment*, portrays inflamed anger at a point of high vulnerability (a loved one's pain) in an unforgettable scene. Her daughter's pain medication is scheduled to be administered at 10:00 a.m. Aurora appears at the desk a few moments past 10:00 a.m. to remind the nurses that it is past time. She encounters two rather disconnected nurses who look up from their charts. One responds, "I was going to give the shot; I will in just a few minutes," and the other nurse responds, "Ma'am, she's not my patient." Aurora begins screaming, "Give my daughter the shot!" Still not getting the response she's looking for, she makes quite a scene, flailing her arms, running around the nurses' desk, screaming repeatedly, "Give my daughter the shot!" Only when a nurse finally rises from behind the nurses' station and gets up to get the shot, does Aurora stop screaming. She straightens her hair and her blouse and murmurs, "Thank you very much."

We can all identify with the distraught mother and predict her outrage as soon as we observe the passive, disconnected response she gets from the staff. The mother's reality and the nurses' reality were worlds apart. That her daughter was in pain was everything to the mother, and the message she received was that the nurses simply didn't understand that. Their disconnection means danger to Aurora; it means more pain for her daughter and that this mother is in it alone. When a family member is grieving and helplessly watching a loved one suffer, asks for help, and encounters disconnected clinicians who do not seem to comprehend the magnitude of the situation to the family member (including a mother's unspoken guilt at all the ways she has failed her daughter in the past), it is a recipe for anger, perhaps even rage or violence.

On a slightly humorous note, sometimes people tell us stories that parallel this one, and they often begin by saying something like, "I pulled a Shirley MacLaine after my brother's surgery . . . he was in such pain and I was out of control . . . ."

It may seem far from justifiable for a family member to react in an out-of-control way, but it is all a matter of perspective. To us, the caregiver, we are one minute late. To her, the patient's terrified family member, we have abandoned her loved one leaving her to suffer.

Another frequent point of high vulnerability is admission for hospitalization. In fast-paced inpatient settings, "one more admit" can be viewed as a source of stress by the staff. Workload has increased, assignments are expanded, and responsibilities may need to be redistributed—all due to one more admit.

It is understandable that "one more admit" sometimes makes clinical staff feel burdened, but that may be because in the frenzy of the shift, an "admit" is not really a person—it's an abstract concept, an obstacle to getting everything done, to experiencing the yearned-for sense of completion of the other care rendered during that shift. If the staff assigned to care for a person during the admission process gives no indication that they are interested in him, the person is more likely to become fearful, wary, and mistrusting. These are all feelings that create the conditions for agitation and anger.

In the frenzy of the shift, an "admit" is not really a person—it's an abstract concept, an obstacle to getting everything done.

Staying Connected in the Face of Anger: "Power Down and Listen"

In the early 1990s, Smith and Hart (1994) studied how medical-surgical nurses managed angry patient interactions. They found that if nurses perceived the anger as a personal attack, they tended to disconnect. Disconnection diverted them from seeking to understand the patient's perspective and experience. Disconnection paved the way for such strategies as taking a time out, blaming the patient, seeking peer support to help ease the nurse's discomfort, and "returning to smooth"—which meant going back to see the patient, but not addressing the anger. "Smoothing" made it possible to go on as though nothing had happened.

The Smith and Hart study also revealed much more effective nurse responses to angry patients, including remaining connected with the patient through the angry episode, wondering about and evaluating the reason for the anger, and perhaps most significantly, not taking it personally.

For the small number of nurses in this study who were able to keep from taking the anger of others personally, a tremendous number of options for dealing with anger were available. Because their inclination was neither to "power up" nor to shut down in the face of anger, their creativity remained, and they could recognize more easily the myriad solutions that presented themselves. The following story, told to us by a workshop participant, illustrates how "powering down" can change a situation dramatically.

Treating the Patient—Not the Anger

Dr. M., the medical director of our hospice program, received a call from Grace, the wife of a patient being cared for in a local hospital. Grace was extremely distressed—crying and begging Dr. M. to admit her husband James to the hospice residence. Grace told Dr. M. that she couldn't bear the way James was being treated at the hospital. He was extremely confused and agitated and at times physically hitting out at caregivers. His agitation was getting worse and the more forceful and restrictive the interventions were, the worse he seemed to get.

Grace knew her husband was dying, and she couldn't bear to see him suffering such assaults on his dignity and humanity in his last days on earth. We didn't take admissions after 3 p.m., and there were other complicating factors, but Dr. M. bypassed all the rules and told Grace she could have James transferred to the hospice residence late that afternoon. They arrived with James on a stretcher. We pulled the covers back and saw that he was in four-point restraints. I immediately took out my scissors and cut the restraints. As I did that, I looked at Grace and saw tears streaming down her face.

James was agitated as we transferred him to the bed, but with Grace's help and comforting voice, he seemed to settle slightly. We pulled four chairs around James' bed to prevent him from falling or crawling out. As he continued to cry out and flail, I asked Grace if she would like to hold James. She immediately crawled into bed with him and cradled him in her arms. James settled instantly. He died three hours later.

The health care team in the hospice residence opened their arms and hearts to Grace and James. Because they saw James as a person, they recognized his anger and confusion as a normal part of his dying process. In the terminal phase of his life, he had become confused, delusional, and fearful. He felt like a small child or a wounded animal, and he flailed and cried. The use of restraints and force exacerbated his fear, isolation, and suffering. The hospice team understood this, so they "powered down." They attuned to Grace and James with compassion and wonder. They palpated the situation, listened to Grace and James, and followed their cues. Because of their ability to listen and see, they were able to find a compassionate, tender solution: Grace held James and comforted him so that he was able to transition out of this world safely and peacefully. By their loving actions, the team provided a foundation for Grace to heal. Grace would always know she protected her husband by advocating for and achieving his transfer and that she was able to be with him and ease his suffering as she held and comforted him in his final hours.

There is, however, always the possibility that anger may escalate into aggressive and even violent behavior. Clinicians need to be attuned to and follow (palpate) angry circumstances by noticing signs of increasing agitation—clenched fists, pacing, threatening movements, significant alterations in voice levels. In less extreme situations the primary caregiver should be certain that the rest of the team knows she is helping a distressed and angry person, and that others on the team are there to back her up should the situation escalate.

Of course the clinician's safety is important. There are threats for which it is best to have security staff on hand. But what might this look like when the principles of the therapeutic relationship are applied?

Dylan Hockett is the director of security for two hospitals in a health care system in Colorado. His philosophy for his security team is that they should be grounded in compassion rather than enforcement (personal communication, November 9, 2011). He says that the majority of security calls in health care are in response to people who are acting out due to feeling overwhelmed, fearful, and powerless to cope with distressing circumstances. It may also be that family dynamics and other external stressors are exacerbated by the illness or crisis. If the security officer enters the scene as "the enforcer," he or she will escalate the situation every time. Hockett believes that people miss the opportunity to provide a healing and supportive intervention by such "powering up."

His ideal scenario is that clinicians who may have called for assistance with an angry patient or family member will think of the security officer as a therapeutic partner, and he's trained his staff to be just that.

In such a scenario it's essential that clinicians remain on the scene and attempt to care for the angry person, knowing that their security partner is at their side; this allows the clinicians to feel safe and able to relax into helping the angry person reach resolution by powering down and listening without fear. Hockett emphasizes that the primary skill required by security personnel when they need to intervene directly, is the ability to connect with and listen to the distressed (angry, aggressive, violent) individual (personal communication, November 9, 2011). The worst-case scenario, according to Hockett, is for the security officers to arrive and the clinical staff to depart the scene, leaving the angry person alone with just the security staff. In that scenario, the angry and distressed person may feel further abandoned and rejected. It also means that the security person, a stranger, needs to begin anew trying to establish connection with an already distraught person. The intervention is less effective in these circumstances.

Hockett uses circle methodology for the security team to meet and reflect on their work. He often begins the circle by inquiring, "What therapeutic action have you taken this past week?" He has been touched by many stories, but one memorable therapeutic action described was that of a security officer who sat on the floor in the emergency room with a distressed child and colored with him in his coloring book—a therapeutic action that helped the child calm down and accept support.

"What therapeutic action have you taken this past week?"

General principles for powering down include:

- Remember that the source of anger is fear, vulnerability, and suffering.

- Powering up escalates tensions and the potential for actual violence; powering down de-escalates them.

- See through the anger to the humanity of the distressed person.

- Wondering about what the expression of anger means to the other helps focus on anger as a symptom rather than personalizing the anger and becoming defensive.

- By following, you encourage the individual to express his anger as you listen, acknowledge, and gain understanding.

- Hold the person in your sturdy care. Anger may be followed by feelings of shame and self-condemnation. Acceptance and compassionate care transcend the situation and re-establish safety.

If patient and family anger are among the hardest things for you to deal with, we invite you to become (unofficially, of course) a patient and family anger specialist. Train yourself to stop and wonder in the face of anger, whether it's directed at you or not. Teach yourself to listen for hints of the patient's back story or prior experience in health care. Attune yourself to your patients as people and see how your experience of their anger changes. Remember that anger is an emotional symptom of distress just as bleeding is a symptom of physiological distress. Anger is a crying out in fear and powerlessness—a crying out for love and connection.

Obstacle Four: The Judging Mind

To judge means to form an opinion or evaluation of another person or circumstance. We usually do this by way of a shorthand method of comparing: right-wrong, good-bad, alike-different, friendly-distant, healthy-sick, crabby-cooperative. Our minds work rapidly, and a big part of what our minds do is to draw conclusions. It's nearly automatic. As we described in our chapter on wondering, Antonio Damasio (1994; 2003) refers to this phenomenon when describing his somatic marker hypothesis. Somatic markers are the stored information that helps us make sense of what we see based on past experiences.

His hypothesis works this way: Let's say I see a squirrel scurrying across the street. What if my mind were incapable of using information about squirrels acquired from years of noticing them? What if I had no capacity to do quick comparisons of this animal with other animals I have known or read about with information stored handily in my brain? I would have absolutely no idea what to expect from this present encounter, much less what to do next about it. I wouldn't know whether to pause and appreciate the cute little thing with the bushy tail or to run frantically to get away from the terrifying little monster! Without somatic markers I would have to start the judging process—essential to daily functioning and survival—all over again with no basis for comparison and no way to reach conclusions.

This, Damasio says, is the problem in mental processing: in daily living, there's simply too much to process if we start every encounter, every decision, every move, as if none of it were familiar. Every day we come across thousands of things that require our attention, assessment, consideration, and response.

Evolution solved this problem—though perhaps imperfectly—by developing somatic markers which enable us to make quick comparisons and to "know" (or rather to assume we know) something about just about everything we encounter. We developed a mental process so rapid that it barely reaches our consciousness, a process by which we project onto our mental screen dozens of scenarios from the past, then link them to the present and the future. That way we know what to do right now and what to do next time. It's a sophisticated, subconscious triage, even faster and more data-filled than the triage that health care workers do every day in the emergency room.

As necessary as this mental processing strategy is, however, it is chock full of inherent problems. First of all, Damasio reports, we rarely store anything in our brains without adding an emotional load—a sort of sidebar containing additional information about how the experience affected us or made us feel at the moment it was happening. Therefore, when we pull up this stored record, the feelings come with the data. If the first time we saw a squirrel we were on a rare and pleasant walk in the woods with Grandpa, our encounter with a squirrel years later will be tinged with pleasant feelings and an absence of fear. But the problem with this emotional loading is clear:

we are at constant risk of misjudging present circumstances based on what we experienced in seemingly similar circumstances we encountered before.

A second problem with this mental strategy is that we human beings are not very good at observing things in purely objective ways. Therefore, when we compare present experience with past experience we encounter more than raw, factual information; we encounter our own biases that were injected into our memory of past events or of people encountered in the past. When a child who lost his first mother—or was abused by her—is approached by a nurturing foster mother, he responds not on the basis of factual information about the new mother. He responds to her as if she fits right in with his perceptions of "mother," based on his experiences with someone by this description from his past. He may avoid her nurturing hugs because his somatic marker suggests that such hugs will soon be followed by hitting or leaving. He may run away for the same reason, or he may hit because the information in his brain says that mothers are dangerous.

This natural but mostly unconscious tendency to draw conclusions based on past events is why we label people. When we refer to a patient as a "frequent flyer," we are simply letting our somatic markers do the work of automatic judging for us. We say, in effect, "Oh, I know all about people like you. I've seen you before. I already know you. I can take a shortcut here. After all, I'm in a hurry. I know just what to expect."

If you're having trouble connecting with this idea of a somatic marker, try this experiment. Notice your "gut reactions" to these labels:

- Conservative
- Fundamentalist
- Demanding
- Liberal
- Drug Seeker
- V.I.P.
- Schizophrenic
- Public Assistance Case
- Drunk
- Narcissistic
- Privileged

Chances are the moment you read each of these labels your mind conducted an instantaneous and subconscious search for data. You may have thought about people you have known or seen portrayed in the media who matched these labels. You may have felt what it was like to be with them or to have cared for them (or to be raised by them or married to them). It is a perfectly natural process and necessary for an efficient existence, but if you are called upon to care for a person who was identified with a label by one of your colleagues—for example, demanding—you might find that your vision of that person would narrow to fit that label.

Labeling, it turns out, changes both the labeler and the labeled. When wondering stops and labeling begins, our behavior toward the one we've labeled changes.

Your openness to the ways this new person failed to match your label could be challenged. You might imagine that you knew enough about her already.

And you know the odd thing? We may actually get something resembling what we predicted we would. Labeling, it turns out, changes both the labeler and the labeled. When wondering stops and labeling begins, our behavior toward the one we've labeled changes. In spite of our contentions to the contrary, the labeled person is no longer truly a person. We begin to respond to the person as if he were the label, and in these instances, it's remarkably common for the labeled person to begin to respond in ways that confirm for us that we were right.

Our tendency to judge, then, is both necessary and automatic, but it is also potentially problematic unless we add wondering. The judging mind that also wonders is a mature mind. It remains curious. It follows. With this mind in gear, we are able to notice our thoughts before we act on them; to scan for and suspend our biases; to avoid labeling (or at least to avoid believing the labels that pop into our minds); to encounter the situation or the person as if they are interesting to us, because we've never really been here, or with this person, before.

Michael's professional world (clinical psychology and counseling) is, unhappily, built on labels. When parents bring their troubled, acting-out child to him, they often seem to want him to label the child. They are often disappointed when he demurs, asking to learn about the etiology of the child's behavior, the story of the child's life, the challenges the child has encountered or is presently contending with.

Parents' impatience arises, understandably, from their hunger for answers, and they imagine that answers will arise from the label. If Billy has "Rufus' Syndrome" (which is completely made up), then his behavior will all be explained, everyone can breathe a sigh of relief that they didn't cause it, and teachers and parents can know just what to do.

The problem is that labels rarely teach us much about a particular child. We pretend they do because it would be so comforting if they did. Then everyone could be fit into this or that box and we would know all about them. But the opposite is true. Labeling usually stops the inquiry. Labeling encourages us to stop being curious. We think we already know, so we're not too interested anymore in the things that would actually help us to understand.

See how your judging mind reacts to this story even before you get to the end. It's nurse Joan Wyjack's remembrance (personal communication, February 27, 2011) of her most challenging patient.

The Painful Trap of "Justified" Judgment

One of my most difficult memories of past patients was a man who has affected my care for each and every patient I have had since that time.

303

He was a life-time prisoner, a crude and rude man out to repulse and alienate everyone he could. He came to us because he had meningitis and they could not manage it at the prison infirmary. We had him for six weeks while he was on antibiotics, and during that time he tested the patience of everyone on the floor. He had an armed guard with him at all times and his hands and feet were shackled to a belly chain which was, in turn, shackled to the bed. I was glad to see him go when his antibiotics were done. I was young—in my mid 20's at the time—and he was intimidating and awful.

Less than four weeks later he came back into the hospital, and after some testing, was diagnosed with advanced cancer. He had very little time to live. He rapidly became demented, unable to make decisions for himself. His body was a war zone of the cancer, swelling, draining, bleeding . . . all while shackled to a bed.

Because of his life and his choices he had no one who would claim him as family, and therefore no one who could make end-of-life decisions for him. He rapidly went downhill while the cuffs bit into his swollen ankles, creating even more physical pain. The state could not issue a Do Not Resuscitate order and neither could his doctors. It was a living hell for him and for those of us who took that trip with him. He endured two full months of this suffering before he passed away. All of that time was spent on our floor. I was there as he passed. It was the first time I had ever experienced a person dying in such an awful and inhumane way—in almost complete isolation from any but the most unavoidable human contact. It hurt so intensely that I could hardly live with it. I did not sleep for days; I could not eat. I felt this pain as intensely as a knife wound in my heart.

After several nights, I finally fell into a restless sleep. I was awakened in a wash of bright light and became aware of a presence. I had to face what had happened, and a single question came to me: What did you do to save this man?

All I could do was cry. I had done nothing but judge him, not even knowing what he had done. I had not seen him as a man, as a human like me, but as an animal who deserved to die. The conviction I felt that night was excruciating. It has forever stayed with me and reminds me to this day that each and every one of us fails in many ways. Who am I to judge?

What did you notice about your own judging mind as you read this story? Did you feel judgment for the dying prisoner? Did you feel judgment for the nurse? Did you feel empathy or compassion for either one? If wondering could have softened anyone's judgment of the dying prisoner, how might those two months have been different for both the prisoner and the clinicians caring for him? Did you feel gratitude for this courageous nurse's willingness to be vulnerable enough to share such a painful personal story? Would you be equally courageous if asked to share your most painful care story? What good may come from sharing and reflecting on stories such as this one?

We are not suggesting that we can do away with our judging mind. It's a part of us. What we're suggesting is that we can choose to pay attention to our thoughts so that we are not ruled by our inner dialogue and driven to habitual and unconscious actions and reactions. We can also choose to recognize others' judgments and consciously decide not to be ruled by them. We can choose not to use language that labels people, such as train wreck, complainer, princess, frequent flyer, or drug seeker. These labels objectify people and create the conditions that move us to automatic judgment. When others use those labels, we can choose to say (without judging the one who has used the label), "Tell me more about what's going on with this person right now." If we're successful in this pursuit, we make way for something new: for encountering this person, at this moment, under these circumstances, in this room, with this family, as altogether fresh and new.

Learning to recognize and suspend our judgments is a mental process that has three practical steps:

1. Mentally shift to a position of neutrality and simply notice your judging thoughts.

2. Mentally place your judgments in a state of suspension like a cartoon thought-bubble that sits silently nearby. The judgments will be there for you if you want them, but they are set aside so they won't interfere with what you are actually seeing and hearing and learning.

3. Mentally release those judging thoughts that are not serving you or others, and consciously open yourself to wondering about the person in front of you right now.

Try this imagery to understand what happens when judgment meets wonder. Imagine a snowball to represent judgment. It's icy and cold, packed tightly together. Now imagine that wonder is a tea kettle full of hot water. If you pour wonder over judgment it melts. Perhaps it's true that judgment "just is," but it is equally true that judgment cannot hold up in the face of wonder.

All of the obstacles to the therapeutic relationship have at least one thing in common: they interfere with our ability to attune to our patients and their families because they stop us from wondering, following, and holding. When we hear at the nurses' station that "We've got a TWF (Turn-Water-Feed) in 312," it is a monumental challenge to overcome the social pressure to accept that insidious labeling. For some, it is an even greater challenge to walk into room 312 and see an actual person. Yet clinicians manage to connect therapeutically with their patients every day despite these obstacles. It's vital to remember that caring and connection can be conveyed in a moment. One touch, one word, the simple act of slowing down—all of these can communicate to a person that she is seen or that he is safe.

Clearly there are some practical things, such as spending five minutes at the patient's side that we can do to save time and cut through the chaos. But the lion's share of what we can do to cut through the chaos is accomplished by reflecting on who we are in relation to the obstacles we encounter and gaining clarity about what is ours to own. Through such self-reflection we strengthen our ability to be more intentional and proactive. If we are clear about our purpose and the importance of the therapeutic relationship to healing and recovery, we will find ways to work with our colleagues to assure that such care is supported and achieved. When we understand the normal responses to illness and crisis, we'll find the ability to stay fully present with those who are suffering, doing what we can to ease the person's pain, fear, anger, and other signs of emotional distress by powering down and listening. Finally, we understand that by becoming more aware of the judging mind, we can suspend judgment and remain more curious, open, accepting, and compassionate.

The Fundamental Obstacle: Compassion Fatigue

No discussion of the obstacles to compassionate, therapeutic care would be complete without addressing the phenomenon of compassion fatigue. This story was told by a nursing director many years ago.

A Moment of Grace

It was 5:15 a.m. when the nursing director walked into the emergency department. She was not expected at that hour of

307

the day and was rather surprised to find the department quiet—in fact it felt almost deserted—and a nurse (Kate) sitting at the reception desk playing solitaire. This nurse's attitude had never been the best, and now she was sitting in public view playing cards. Kate did not look up, but apathetically turned over one card after another.

By the director's own admission, it was nothing short of a miracle, a moment of grace, that stopped her from rushing to judgment and led her instead to attune to Kate and realize that something significant was going on.

The director walked around the desk and pulled a chair up beside Kate. Kate stared down at the cards and said nothing. The director placed her hand on Kate's shoulder and asked, "What's going on?" With that, silent tears streamed down Kate's face and she shook her head side to side. "What is it, Kate?" The director held her as Kate slumped against her. They sat like that for some minutes.

Finally, Kate said that she was trying to hold herself together. An hour earlier, a 35-year-old man had been taken to the OR after being brought in to the ED. He'd been standing by the side of the road and was hit by a truck that amputated his left leg at the hip. The team had worked for hours to stabilize him and get him to the OR. She and another nurse had stayed behind to clean the blood from the room while other members of the team transported the man to surgery. Kate had been an ED nurse for two years and thought she had seen a lot, but this night, this man, and the horror of this accident felt like more than she could bear.

Exposure to a traumatic event such as this one, as well as the more subtle and chronic witnessing of the pain and suffering of others, can take a significant emotional toll on caregivers. Add to that the chaos, time constraints, and high volume of patients and families, and we have a recipe for burnout and compassion fatigue.

Compassion fatigue was originally named as a specific concept in 1992 by Carla Joinson. She described compassion fatigue as chronic burnout eventually resulting in nurses losing their compassion and their ability to empathize with others. According to Joinson, caregivers who are worn down by daily exposure to hospital emergencies and patient suffering become disconnected from the people around them. Vicarious traumatization occurs when one is exposed to extreme traumatic injuries and becomes overwhelmed or emotionally incapacitated by the images (Figley, 1995).

Pfifferling and Gilley (2000) describe compassion fatigue with this illustration of a family practice physician:

> Andy had always been an energetic and dedicated family physician. Now, at 38, he's tired, cynical and lonely. He's angry at the health care system for forcing him to see more patients in less time and annoyed with his patients for what he perceives to be their increasingly demanding natures. Although his relationships with his patients once thrived, they no longer seem to give him the same satisfaction. Even talking to his wife, who's always been a supportive partner, has not relieved his feelings of intense isolation. (p. 39)

Some who have experienced compassion fatigue describe it as "being sucked into a vortex that pulls them slowly downward" (Pfifferling & Gilley, 2000, p. 39). Health care professionals describe the intense demands of the health care environment as contributing to compassion fatigue, including the requirement to see more patients in circumscribed periods of time and learning new technologies while fulfilling their own high standards of care under circumstances of reduced autonomy and regulation. Additionally (and we believe quite significantly) some grieve the loss of relationships they once shared with their patients. Pfifferling and Gilley note that when family physicians had time to connect with their patients as human beings, they experienced less compassion fatigue because they received "the replenishment they needed to cope with the stressors of practicing medicine" (2000, p. 40). It seems that it isn't just patients who suffer when we don't take the time to build connection with them; clinicians may be suffering from repeated encounters with individuals in which only surface-level connections are being established. They lose their connection with people and it cannot help but follow that they lose their connection with the meaning of their work.

For information on identifying compassion fatigue in individuals and organizations, please see Appendix F on page 404.

How Lack of Human Connection Contributes to Compassion Fatigue

Kristen Swanson, professor and theorist renowned for the Swanson Theory of Caring, proposes that burnout and compassion fatigue result from "loss of integrity" (personal communication, November, 1990). In Swanson's research on nurse caring (2007), she found that ". . . compromising quality of care for quantity of care can only go on so long before nurses (individually or collectively) give up hope and lose their capacity to practice from a position of compassion" (p. 506).

Put succinctly, when we fail to see our work as caring for people and instead think of our work in terms of functions to carry out, we lose our integrity and we burn out. This observation is confirmed by scholars in the fields of physical therapy and nursing. They find that disconnection from our human capacity for compassion and the associated values that call us into this humanitarian field lead to burnout and loss of spirit (Schuster, Nelson, & Quisling, 1984; Watson, 2005).

According to Swanson (1990), there are four aspects of clinical practice, two relational (role attachment and caring) and two instrumental (managing responsibilities and preventing poor outcomes), which must remain in balance if we are to maintain our integrity as clinicians. Swanson's identification of these four aspects gives us insight into what happens when clinicians feel disconnected from the people in their care as well as from their colleagues. When the instrumental elements of care dominate our practice, we become estranged from the humans around us, we feel isolated, and we lose our connection to the purpose of our work and the reason we went into health care in the first place.

As you read these descriptions of the four aspects of clinical practice outlined by Swanson, consider how much each aspect influences your practice and whether you're able to maintain a balance among them.

Relational

1. **Role Attachment:** As people enter the health care professions, they form an attachment to their professional role as they define it. Their role identity typically includes being a highly competent clinician who forms therapeutic relationships with those in their care. When clinicians work within cultures in which establishing and nurturing therapeutic relationships with patients and their families is not supported, those clinicians begin to feel disconnected from the reason they entered the profession.

2. **Caring:** Caring is frequently described as the essence of professional practice and is understood to be a fundamental component for the provision of humane, compassionate, quality patient care. When clinicians fail to connect honestly, authentically, and

spontaneously with patients, families, and colleagues, they find themselves dispirited; they lose their sense of purpose in their work. Organizational cultures that lack systems to support the clinician-patient relationship may be among the most common causes of compassion fatigue.

Instrumental

3. **Managing Responsibilities:** Professional licensure and employment within health care organizations are contingent upon a clinician's willingness to accept specific responsibilities for the provision of care. These responsibilities must be fulfilled. When clinicians perceive that they are falling short of fulfilling their responsibilities, they experience stress.

4. **Preventing Poor Outcomes:** Concomitant with responsibility acceptance is accountability for safe care. This means that each clinician is proficient in the provision of care and vigilant in preventing harm. When clinicians are unable to prevent poor outcomes and when their work life does not include adequate reflection (ideally with others) about how to prevent those outcomes in the future, they risk chronic stress and burnout.

Swanson (1990) points out that far too often the pressure to tend to the management of responsibilities and prevention of poor outcomes leads clinicians to grieve the loss of the human connection that accompanies the expression of both role attachment and caring.

Whenever we meet clinicians who are feeling dispirited in their work, we consistently find that they are feeling disconnected from people. Almost as frequently, we see them attributing that disconnection to the lack of time to build therapeutic relationships. But it bears noting that caring and feeling connected are internal processes, both of which typically also become visible to patients and their families. A clinician can nurture his connection to his role (what Swanson calls his role attachment) through nothing more than centering himself often throughout his day, remembering his purpose, and consciously intending to connect on a human-to-human basis with everyone he encounters.

Whenever we meet clinicians who are feeling dispirited in their work, we consistently find that they are feeling disconnected from people.

It's obvious that role attachment and caring are expressions of human connection, but it's equally true that managing responsibility and preventing poor outcomes require human connection in order to be tended to effectively. In a worst-case scenario, a blood draw is an entirely instrumental task requiring nothing more than a connection between a clinician, an instrument, and a vein. In a best-case scenario, a blood draw is an encounter between two people who see each other as people and in which the brief but vital connection formed between these two people ensures that blood is drawn with as little worry or discomfort as possible.

The admission of a patient and transmission of information about a patient don't take longer if questions are asked and the patient's cues are followed. In fact we find that time is saved in the long run when we connect with our patients as people.

The Perspective that Keeps Compassion Fatigue at Bay

The therapeutic practices of wondering, following, and holding, when practiced within a container of presence and attunement, keep clinicians focused on the newness, complexity, and vulnerability of the people in our care. When these practices are employed consistently, they lead us to purposefully attune ourselves to every person and every situation we encounter. When we are willing to wonder about each person, we lose the sense of repetitiveness about our work. Indeed, it's never the case that we fill out the same form again and again; if it's about the unique person, not the form, there is nothing repetitive about what we do.

There is an old story about two men in the 16th century who work long, grueling hours side by side every day. One is asked what he does to earn his living, and he replies that he is a brick layer. The other, who is quite obviously doing exactly the same physical work, is asked what he does for a living, and he says that he is building a great cathedral to honor God. They do the same work, technically speaking, but one of these men brings wonder and attunement (and so much more) to every moment of it. Do you imagine that one of these men will tire more quickly than the other?

Reflection is key to the internal decision that each of us makes about who we are in our work. We can see ourselves as the unthanked servants of people who sometimes show little regard for what we're offering and sometimes show outright contempt for it. Or we can see ourselves as individuals who are committed to building something beautiful—an authentic, spontaneous human relationship—over and over, each time in unique ways.

Our commitment to our work is likely to ebb and flow throughout our lives. There will be many who theorize about why this happens and many who offer truly valuable solutions. We believe, however, that the solutions that work will always be those that lead us back to authentic human connection.

Summary of Key Thoughts

- When this question is asked of clinicians: "What personal factors or external stressors challenge your ability or the ability of your colleagues to establish a therapeutic relationship with patients and families?" these are the three most frequent answers: 1) time constraints and conflicting priorities; 2) fast-paced, complicated environments; 3) the tendency to judge or discount people perceived as demanding and difficult.

- When this question is asked of clinicians: "What are the most challenging patient and family interactions for you?" these are the three most frequent answers: 1) highly critical or demanding patients and families; 2) families who appear uncaring or potentially harmful to patients; 3) patients or families projecting anger verbally and/or physically toward the caregiver.

- All of the obstacles to the therapeutic relationship have at least one thing in common: they interfere with our ability to attune to our patients and their families as they stop us from wondering, following, and holding.

- When people are highly self-differentiated they have what psychologists term an internal locus of control. Their sense of what to do in any given moment comes from inside; it is not based on what they think others might want them to do.

- People with an external locus of control (those who are less self-differentiated) perceive that others determine in what ways they are expected or permitted to act.

- When we move our focus into the Circle of Influence we are in a position to take action which creates a positive forward movement. In this circle, we are far more self-differentiated.

- One of the key predictors of quality patient care is the commitment of a team of clinicians who are devoted to being there for each other in service to their patients and families.

- When a Code Compassion is called, a community of caregivers knows exactly what to do in order to assure that other patients are not neglected while one colleague focuses on a patient needing an extra dose of therapeutic attention.

- The phenomenon of entrainment suggests that we may get pulled into the too-fast rhythm of what is going on around us. The routine of hand washing between patients can be used as a cue to downshift and be more attuned to the rhythm of the patient.

- The literature on anger and illness consistently correlates the root cause of anger with fear and vulnerability.

- A "top five" list of human responses to illness and/or crisis are:
  1. fear,
  2. grief and loss,
  3. pain (physical, emotional, and spiritual),
  4. difficulty coping, and
  5. powerlessness.

- When we are deep in wonder about another person's expression of anger, we cannot be adversely affected by his anger.

- There are four identifiable patterns that can exacerbate fear and powerlessness and engender anger in patients and their family members:

  1. The patient's and family's established pattern of emotional response

  2. The patient's and family's back story

  3. The patient's and family's previous experience of safety and care in health care settings

  4. Points of high vulnerability for the patient and family during the care episode

- Patterns of emotional response cannot be counted on to follow the rules of reason and logic. Because our patterns of emotional response were formed long ago, many of them were formed while we were too young to be rational; it's not uncommon for people to regress when they're in distress (Strain, 1979).

- By wondering about an individual's back story (whether we discover it or not), we become more able to attune, follow, and hold the other with compassion, which facilitates the release of anger and opens up the possibility of trust, connection, and healing.

- There are predictable points in a care experience that potentially increase anxiety or heighten a person's feelings of fear and powerlessness.

- In the frenzy of the shift, we need to remember that every new "admit" is a human being, not an obstacle to getting everything done or leaving work on time.

- Our tendency to judge is necessary and automatic, but it is also potentially problematic unless we add wondering. The judging mind that also wonders is a mature mind. It remains curious. It follows. It continues to learn.

- Labeling usually hinders (or stops) our inquiry. We think we already know, so we're not too interested anymore in the things that would actually help us to understand.

- Exposure to a traumatic event, as well as the more subtle and chronic exposure of witnessing the pain and suffering of others over time, can take a significant emotional toll on caregivers. Add to that the chaos, time constraints, and volumes of patients and families, and we have a recipe for burnout and compassion fatigue.

- When the instrumental elements of care are permitted to dominate our practice, we become estranged from the humans around us, we feel isolated, and we lose our connection to the purpose of our work and the reason we went into health care in the first place.

- The therapeutic practices of wondering, following, and holding, when practiced within a container of presence and attunement, keep clinicians focused on the newness, complexity, and vulnerability of the people in our care.

Reflection

- An exemplar stated the following about the importance of her own daily self-talk: "My mantra is to think 'we' instead of 'me.' When I think 'we' I use connecting language and behave in connecting ways." In your experience, to what extent do you think of yourself as an individual working alone, and to what extent do you think of yourself as part of an interdependent team? What might your own self-talk indicate about how connected you feel to the people on your team?

- What is more challenging for you to be with: a patient's depression and withdrawal or a patient's overt expression of anger? Why do you think that one may challenge you more than the other?

- When Dr. H. spent time with the "meanest patient in the world" he was not invested in an outcome. In what specific ways might his "lack of agenda" have helped Dr. H.? What would it take for you to be in a similar state of mind with a patient who was expressing overt anger or profound depression?

- Marie Manthey says: "The 'closed door of power' (personal or professional) only opens when I actively accept responsibility for myself and my own actions 100% of the time." What does this mean to you?

- Consider the following statement: "I realize that in those times when I accept responsibility, it is impossible for me to feel victimized. Conversely, in those times when I do not accept responsibility, I feel victimized." In your experience, what is the correlation between responsibility acceptance and ceasing to feel victimized?

- Consider the following quote from an exemplar: "I practice self-awareness and notice and suspend my own judgments; I know what my triggers are, and noticing them helps me suspend judgment. I also ask for help from trusted team members. We have worked hard to build a culture that fosters self-awareness and team support." What thoughts do you have about this person's perspective? What does it mean to you to have "a culture of self-awareness and team support"? What would it take for you and your team to build such a culture?

- Transitions are times of vulnerability for patients, and emotional regression sometimes happens when we're extremely vulnerable. On a pediatric wing, we might see easily that a 7-year-old will regress to a 2-year-old's behavior when vulnerable, and we may also see that a 37-year-old might regress to the 7-year-old's behavior under difficult circumstances. What has your experience been with patients who show regressive behavior? When you experience this behavior, what might help you remember to wonder instead of reacting in another way?

- This chapter talked about a situation in which a team was supportive enough of each other that they were able to call a Code Compassion when a patient or family member was in extra need of therapeutic attention. Would Code Compassion be easy or difficult to fit into your current team culture? What would it take to prepare your team to establish Code Compassion as a norm within your work culture?

- What are your thoughts about this statement? "A team that is dedicated to high-quality therapeutic care will cultivate peer consultations as a norm." What would it take to cultivate peer consultations as a norm in your practice and environment?

- What do you think about the statement: "When we label our patients, we're no longer holding them; our devotion to them is gone." What has been your experience with labeling?

- We talked about the importance of understanding that every patient and family member has a back story. Why might it be important to remember that our team members have back stories too? What might their back stories have to do with how easy or difficult it is for them to collaborate or to stay fully present with those who are suffering or to remember to take care of their own physical and emotional needs? How might understanding your team members' back stories help you to work better with them?

- Ask yourself: How am I relating to my colleagues? Are there people I'm excited to work with and others I dread working with? In my relationships with my colleagues, what is within my sphere of influence to change? What are one or two of my own behaviors that I want to change to improve team relationships?

- Consider this statement: "When we fail to see our work as caring for people, and instead think of our work in terms of tasks to carry out, we lose our integrity and we burn out." What does this mean to you and your practice? What, if anything, do you want to change to achieve greater balance between the relational and instrumental aspects of your work?

- Complete the individual and organizational compassion fatigue assessment in Appendix F on page 404. Reflect on your results with a group of colleagues. What are the implications of your current level of compassion fatigue for your own health and well-being and for the health of your team? What are one or two actions that will help you take better care of yourself and each other?

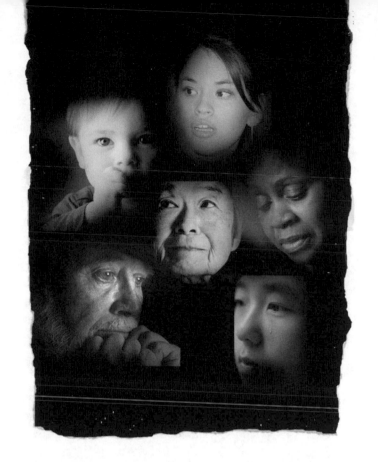

Chapter Seven

Reflective Practice:
The Means by Which Learning
Becomes Permanent

The mind, once expanded to the dimensions of larger ideas, never returns to its original size.

—OLIVER WENDELL HOLMES, SR., PHYSICIAN AND POET

Wisdom begins in wonder.

—SOCRATES

The couple stands at the back door of their house, looking through the screen at the stranger riding away on his white stallion.

"Who was that masked man, Martha?"

"Why George, that was the Lone Ranger!"

How strange. Even on a Saturday morning western, every episode ended with reflection. In the past half-hour, people's lives had been affected by this handsome stranger in the black mask who came out of nowhere to save, defend, uplift, and energize. No one was the same after this man came to town (and then left just as quickly) inspiring awe, envy, rage, relief, and fear.

So folks had to reflect. They didn't just go back to whatever they were doing before the mystery man's arrival. They stopped. They got quiet. They wondered about what had just happened. They tried to find an explanation for it all. As best they could, they reflected. It seemed as though they had to.

"Who was that masked man, Martha?"

"Why George, that was the Lone Ranger!"

And with that, they were able to go back to work.

We seem to be built with both the need to reflect on the important things in our lives and the facility to do just that. The only thing standing in our way is a willingness to let ourselves do what we would naturally do under less hurried circumstances.

It isn't a chore. It isn't an add-on to what we are already obligated to do in our lives. Reflection is the thing that helps it all make sense. It's the thing that helps us incorporate experience, and as a result, learn much more quickly from it. It's the thing that helps us to avoid repeating mistakes. It's the thing that improves our efficiency and our efficacy while allowing us to be so present in each moment that people say our work appears to come naturally to us.

But why can't we just do our jobs?

Did anyone mention during our educational preparation that we would have to be aware of ourselves at all times, noticing not only our instrumental performance and its impact on the patient's body, but also our presence and its impact on the totality of the patient?

Reflection turns out to be one of our most important responsibilities. It also turns out to be one of the things that separates us from technicians. We don't just *do*. We do, we notice our doing, we consider what we did, and we learn from what we did, so that our next doing is informed by past doing. All the while, we think about the context of our doing and we modify our doing in response to that context. Meanwhile we are continuously gathering information from the patient about the meaning and impact of our doing.

In short, we are obligated to reflect automatically on ourselves, on our patients, and on our work, as if such reflection were as important as the acts we are reflecting upon—which, as it turns out, it is.

But why? And when do we have time for this?

Remember when we hadn't learned yet about hand washing in hospitals? We kept noticing things (people getting sicker in the hospital than they had been at home, people getting strange infections while in our care), and we kept fixing things, treating symptoms of whatever illness manifested. It was only when we stepped back and reflected on our practices, talked with people inside and outside of our individual institutions, and considered the possibilities, that something altogether new and unbelievably time-saving, money-saving, reputation-enhancing, and efficient, dawned on us. We had something on our bodies that was infecting people, and we could wash it off before we touched them. Hand washing became the norm, and fewer people got iatrogenic illnesses. It took a few moments to wash properly, but it saved us thousands of moments in the long run.

Reflection works the same way: it takes a few moments to do it properly, but it saves us from making the same mistakes and miscalculations over and over again as well as saving us lots of heartache and frustration.

Reflection is also what transforms wondering, following, and holding from a way of thinking and a way of acting into a way of being.

Reflective Practice is a Pathway to Professional Mastery

The participants in our workshops are highly skilled clinical professionals with years of experience in practice. At the beginning of each workshop, we ask the participants what would make this workshop a success for them—what would make it worth their valuable investment of time and energy. The answer is invariably the same: "I want to learn skills that I can apply in my practice—something new that will help me relate more effectively with my patients and becomes a permanent part of my practice." In other words, people are seeking a way to hold on to and deepen new learning and insights, but their prior experience has been that new learning is often temporary. They describe leaving a great workshop excited about what they've learned, then returning to work and immediately losing what they learned as they get caught up in the routines and habits of their often chaotic work cultures. Participants are hoping it will be different this time. The question is, what does it take for new learning to be integrated and actually put into practice?

Russell Ackoff (1989), an organizational theorist, professor, and pioneer in the field of systems thinking and management science, offers a theoretical framework that helps us understand why some learning is not integrated and "goes in one ear and out the other," while other learning becomes profoundly meaningful to us, sticking with us for life, permanently changing our way of thinking or behaving.

According to Ackoff it is possible for learning to progress from academic ideas to practical application; from temporary data and information to permanent knowledge and understanding; from superficial information to deep understanding and wisdom. Ackoff describes the progression of learning through five levels:

1. Data: factual information or figures

2. Information: data that are connected to something relevant to us; answers the questions who, what, and when

3. Knowledge: application of information; answers the question how

4. Understanding: appreciation of why

5. Wisdom: evaluated and integrated understanding

This progression from data to wisdom, however, is not automatic. We propose that what moves us through this progression is reflection. Reflective practice allows us to take in new learning, apply it, and assess whether the way we've applied it is the best or most effective way. It allows us to continually refine our understanding and to eventually integrate our new learning into our lives. It's exactly what our workshop participants are asking for. The relationship between reflection and the learning progression is illustrated in Figure 7.1 below.

If specific facts and figures are not relevant to us, we forget them quickly. They become relevant for us when we begin to "connect the dots," relating the facts and figures to a *who*, a *what*, and/or a *when*. When we add these dimensions to data, they're transformed into useful information. When we begin to apply what we've learned, we discover *how* this new information works in our own practice and how it relates to things we already know. We begin to transform information into practical knowledge that is accessible and applicable in our daily work. At this point, we're likely to hold onto our new learning at least for a while. If we stop here, perhaps hearing ourselves say, "I already know that," we interrupt our progression to deeper understanding and wisdom. It's through reflection that we continue to synthesize, refine, and integrate our learning so that knowledge is transformed into a permanent way of thinking and understanding.

FIGURE 7.1: Learning Pathway

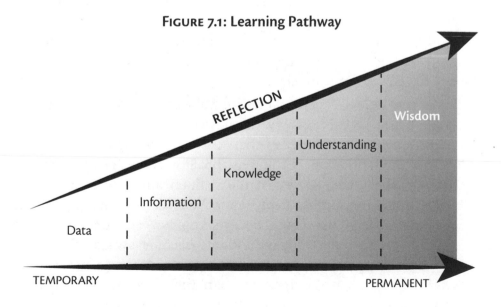

329

If our goal is to have permanent access to the information, knowledge, understanding, and wisdom that we recognize as valuable, we have to go the distance, putting time and intention into applying new concepts in our lives and reflecting on what we're learning. So when our workshop participants ask how they can retain this new knowledge permanently, our answer is: through application and reflection.

One example of how learning progresses through group reflection is seen when participants in our workshops consider the norm or habit of labeling patients and families. We ask whether such labeling interferes with the clinician's ability to attune, wonder, follow, and hold those in their care. Most of the participants have an opinion about labeling, as they already have practical experience and knowledge on the subject. Some acknowledge that labels affect their perception of the person and stimulate surface assumptions that can interfere with their relationship, while others maintain that labels do not affect their ability to see their patients as people, contending that the label simply helps them know what their workload will be like when caring for the labeled patient. They see labeling as a harmless communication shortcut. Still others acknowledge that they find the labels funny and admit that they haven't given it much thought beyond that.

As we reflect together on the subject of labeling, some people begin to shift visibly in their thinking, while others remain quiet and then reveal their insights during the closing circle of the workshop. "I thought that just because *I* could see through labels, they were harmless, but I am now aware of how my labeling might affect how others see the patient, and how the labels I use could be a 'setup' for all concerned." Through group reflection, individuals become aware of how labeling affects others and eventually why labeling has the potential to be more damaging than they'd realized. In the closing circle, some participants verbally commit to discontinue labeling in their practice. Over time (unless something causes them to doubt this learning) these individuals will integrate this knowledge and understanding into their practice, and their practice will be permanently altered.

According to Donald Schön (1987), a pioneer in reflective learning, the instrumental aspects of any professional discipline are most highly valued as the true professional paradigm. The instrumental elements of a profession are taught through the lens of "technical rationality," an educational methodology built on the assumption that "practitioners are instrumental problem solvers who select technical means best suited to particular purposes," and that they solve problems "by applying theory and technique derived from ... preferably scientific knowledge" (pp. 3-4).

The instrumental aspects of our practice are highly conducive to algorithms and protocols and are frequently taught and learned through lecture, application, and observation in practice. There is a right and a wrong way for many of the instrumental skills of our professions to be performed, and these skills can usually be observed and measured.

Schön proposes that if we are overly attached to technical rationality as the only professional paradigm, we will likely miss the richness and value that reflective practice will bring to the "artistry" of our profession. Reflection helps us to notice and then address those elements of our practice that defy predictability and technique. Reflection allows us to continuously learn, refine, become clear, notice variations, and gain in wisdom.

There are no clear-cut right answers or rules to guide us when we are in the "swampy lowland where messy, confusing problems defy technical solution[s]" (Schön, 1987, p. 3). We must navigate these lowlands by seeking greater understanding and wisdom, which are often anything but clear. The relational aspect of our practice is by nature elusive, complex, even mysterious. It's as unpredictable and confounding as the variety of people and circumstances we encounter. There are no algorithms to direct us and no rules that will work every time. What works one time with one person may fail completely with another. While this can indeed be quite challenging for those of us who prefer to work quickly and fix the problem, what we know is that quick fixes rarely resolve issues of deep human concern.

Consider this actual case which illustrates what clinical practice can be like in the swampy lowlands where answers are anything but easy: A baby shrieks for the first seven months of his life. No one is getting any sleep. The parents are utterly depleted. No one has "lost it" yet, but in these situations the possibility of abuse lurks not far around the next bend. The baby is examined over and over. Doctors and nurses test count-less hypotheses about what in the world is the matter with this screaming infant. Medications to ease what they think is physical pain produce no results.

Quick fixes rarely resolve issues of deep human concern.

Finally the beleaguered parents drag themselves to a specialist whose contribution was only to help them reflect. As the three collaborators sat together wondering, the parents happened to mention the child's birth. He was past his due date; his mother was in labor, but things were not progressing. Her dilation stopped at 4 cm, and her original plan for natural childbirth went right out the window. The pain was more than she could bear, and she wanted this baby out! One epidural—then two, then three—did little except immobilize the lower half of her body. Eventually the baby's head crowned enough to use the vacuum extractor. When that was insufficient, forceps were applied, twisting and turning the baby's body. Finally, out he came, screaming, and he did not stop.

Could it be that this baby was still suffering from that extraordinarily difficult birth seven months later? Could it be that he somehow remembered this struggle? Surely this one traumatic experience had nothing to do with his unceasing shriek . . .

That's the thing about reflection: It doesn't necessarily produce perfect answers. It may just produce novel perspectives, an alternative idea, a new way to approach a situation in which nothing else has been working. They didn't have to know for certain, in order to try something novel that came to light through refection.

These desperate parents laid their baby on the floor, hovered over him, and began to tell him how sorry they were. He stopped momentarily and made direct eye contact with his mother. She was startled by this response and kept talking softly to her baby, joined by the father: "You must have hurt so much. You must have wondered why people were doing those things to you. You must have wondered where your mommy was or why your daddy didn't make them stop. Do you know that you're safe now? No one is going to have to do any of those things to you again. We are so sorry that the beginning of your life was so painful."

They went on this way for nearly an hour, transfixed by his eye contact, astonished at the sudden quiet.

The screaming stopped, and it did not return.

Did this reflection and the resulting conversation with the baby take too long? Surely these parents would have been justified in saying that there was simply no time—and no energy—for an entire hour of reflection and acting on that reflection. Yet it was the only thing that actually *gave* them time because it helped them solve the problem at its source.

No one knows exactly why this reflective intervention shifted the situation, and it certainly should stir us to wonder. Was it the parents' gentle attunement with the child? Was it the compassion that helped this baby feel held—truly held, perhaps for the first time? Maybe the baby felt seen for the first time and felt his suffering acknowledged. The cessation of fear and desperation in the parents may have allowed them to really attune to their baby for the first time, relaxing their own repressed guilt about the baby's birth. None of this is conclusively knowable, but we know it was clearly worth reflecting on because the baby's shrieking stopped in one evening.

It happens every day in health care that we notice a problem long before its source is evident. We treat what we see first. The man with clogged arteries gets either a stent or surgery, but we know not to stop there, because we then have to wonder about the source of his problem. He is sent to rehab—not just for the rehabilitation itself, but also for the guided reflection that will happen there: reflection on his eating, exercise, lifestyle, and the stress factors that may have caused the problem in the first place.

What would it take for you, in your busy practice, to use reflection as if it were as important as any other tool in your collection? What would it be like to approach each patient as if she were unique, to approach every challenging situation with flexibility and curiosity? What difference would it make on your unit if it was an everyday occurrence for clinicians to reflect on what works best for Mrs. Holt in 321, on how each staff member is doing after the death of the child who had been on the unit for the past two months, or on what went wrong and what went right with the care of the man with the very fearful wife?

This book has offered you tools for building relationships with your patients that will significantly enhance the efficacy of your care, improve your patients' follow-through on the care plan, ease tensions on your unit, and dramatically improve your patients' satisfaction with your care and with your institution. None of it will work for long, however, without a companion capacity to reflect.

We all run out of energy sooner or later unless we take the time to reflect on who we are, why we're here, and what, if anything, we need to do differently in order for us to live and work with meaning, efficacy, and purpose. We will move away from the sort of practices described in this book if we don't include in the formula some time to reflect on what we're doing, why we're doing it, and what our intentions are for the patients, family members, or team members we encounter. Reflection can be as simple as taking a moment to center ourselves before entering a room so that we are mindful of who this person is, what we're here for, and what's going on for this person right now. Reflective practice is a discipline that moves us to greater understanding and mastery of our practice as individuals and as a team.

Why Vulnerability is Necessary for Reflection

A key factor in our ability to reflect is whether we have learned to embrace our own emotional vulnerability. Assess yourself using these questions:

- Can I look objectively at my own practice? Am I open to learning new things?

- If I discover that I've made a mistake, can I survive the fact that I am flawed? Can I learn from it? Can I forgive myself? Can I move on?

- Can I imagine that understanding what contributed to my actions may improve my practice in the future?

- Do I lapse into shame when I have made a mistake, saying not, "I made a mistake" but rather, "I am a mistake"? (Brown, 2012).

Reflection challenges us to move beyond our most comfortable conclusions. It requires a vulnerability that allows us to risk being wrong, to operate without the net of scientific certainty, and to walk into a room with intelligent ignorance.

A key factor in our ability to reflect is whether we have learned to embrace our own emotional vulnerability.

In our professional lives, it's far more comfortable for us to know than to not know. Fortunately, however, the sort of vulnerability that allows for reflection accepts that not knowing is quite survivable, and in fact can lead to our having more to give both personally and professionally.

It would be rare that someone in any setting would allow herself to be completely vulnerable. In practice, when people choose to be vulnerable, they typically do it in a measured way. I may say in a group setting that I'm going to make myself vulnerable, and what that means to me will vary significantly from what it means to someone else. Perhaps it means that I'm going to be courageous in speaking my truth about what I see happening in my own practice, but I may still be guarded about revealing what's going on in the organization I work in. This is an important reality for any clinician to reflect on. Take a moment now to locate the boundaries you've created around your own vulnerability, using these questions:

- What are the things I'm willing to be open, honest, and vulnerable about? What are the topics or circumstances about which I am more guarded?

- On what topics do I choose to monitor my vulnerability or to have careful boundaries? Why might I continue to keep my boundaries? Why is it important to me to have the boundaries I have?

- What would it take for me to be more vulnerable (unguarded) when discussing topics that are uncomfortable for me? What difference might vulnerability make in my practice?

- Am I a safe person for others to be vulnerable with in a group setting? What could I change in order to help others feel more comfortable being vulnerable with me?

Chris Argyris, in his book *Teaching Smart People How to Learn* (2008), writes that reflection enables professionals to continue to learn and develop in their fields. He also notes, however, that high-performing, well-educated professionals are often hobbled in their learning by their difficulty in admitting that they may not already know something. According to Argyris, such highly educated people tend to believe that they have a professional responsibility to "already know" and that their job is to offer their skills and intelligence.

Argyris describes his own experience of reflection with a group of high-performing professionals as proceeding well at first. The participants seemed highly motivated to learn and seek improvement, until the reflection turned to their own performance within the organization. It was there that something went wrong. Argyris reports:

> It wasn't a matter of bad attitude. The professionals' commitment to excellence was genuine, and the vision of the company was clear. Nevertheless, continuous improvement did not persist.... What happened? The professionals began to feel embarrassed. They were threatened by the prospect of critically examining their own role in the organization....The idea that their performance might not be at its best made them feel guilty.
>
> Far from being a catalyst for real change, such feelings caused most to react defensively. They projected the blame for any problems away from themselves and onto what they said were unclear goals, insensitive and unfair leaders, and stupid clients. (pp. 10-11)

The high intelligence of such professionals endows them with the potential to benefit significantly from the insights gleaned from reflective practice, but it's their very intelligence, not to mention the perfectionism and sense of obligation to be high performers that often accompanies intelligence, which makes them resist using reflection as a catalyst for change. Argyris' premise is that the barrier to reflecting on one's own performance is embarrassment about not knowing or not being good enough. What would it take for us to allow ourselves to let in information that may challenge the usual way we do things? Can we be vulnerable enough and self-forgiving enough to welcome and enjoy the possibilities that come from accepting the challenge to think and practice differently?

Interestingly, the kind of vulnerability we're talking about celebrates our ability to admit that we may have something new to learn and that our wisdom comes from not thinking we have to know it all. This kind of vulnerability is receptive. It invites input. It is curious. It not only allows novelty, it also opens the door wide for new ways of looking at a situation and unexpected ways of addressing a problem.

We are capable of real reflection when we're not terrified that we will be "found out" to have missed something, to have acted improperly, not to have thought of everything. Through reflection we are able to discover our mistakes and repair them. Reflection helps us move beyond habitual patterns to a more mindful practice that facilitates our ability to be therapeutic and responsive to the unique person in front of us right now. It is through reflection that we discover new ways and new possibilities which can lead to exciting breakthroughs in the mastery of our practice.

It seems that every story has potential to provide insights into what went right and what went wrong. Every story of human interaction has potential to expand our knowledge and deepen our understanding about relationships.

We recently heard a story about a nurse who was able to calm a psychiatric patient after a team of people had tried without success to do so.

What Did Tracy Do?

None of us could figure out how Tracy did it. There were at least six of us surrounding Mr. A. He had become increasingly agitated and combative. He was refusing his medications and threatening the staff. We had called security to assist, and we were about to take action to forcibly restrain him.

Then Tracy walked into the room, called him by name, and sat down next to him. She took his hand, knelt in front of him so she was looking him in the eyes, and spoke softly to him. Mr. A. quieted almost immediately. Within a few minutes, he agreed to take his medication and said he did not want to be restrained and would cooperate.

Perhaps it's because Tracy knew him? I tell you, it was something to see.

Unfortunately, that's where the story ended. When we asked whether the team debriefed afterward—whether they'd spent time reflecting on what happened—we learned that they had not. There wasn't enough time, we were told. They were left wondering about what worked, what didn't work, and why, without gaining tangible insights that would have surfaced through reflection. What were the others doing that escalated the patient's distress? What did Tracy do that created such a connection with Mr. A.? Why did Tracy approach Mr. A. so gently when he was so out of control? What was she thinking? Why wasn't she afraid? And perhaps most importantly, what can we learn from Tracy's thinking and actions that will help us in similar situations? If something worked while so many other things failed, wouldn't we want to know everything there was to know about it?

In health care, we are accustomed to reflecting on what worked and what didn't work when we have sentinel events. We are less accustomed to reflecting on everyday practices, but there is great value in looking at a situation in which something has worked unexpectedly. It feels like an opportunity was missed here.

It's possible, of course, that in our analysis we would discover that Tracy did nothing particularly special. Perhaps it was simply that she and Mr. A. had connected previously in a meaningful way that meant he could trust her enough to quiet down and open up. Certainly that, in and of itself, is good information. It's also possible that we would discover something unique and surprising about what Tracy said or did to de-escalate the difficult emotions Mr. A. was suffering with. Perhaps we would discover principles that would help guide us in the next difficult situation.

There is great value in looking at a situation in which something has worked unexpectedly.

Only reflection can get us to that understanding, and such reflection requires us to be curious and to be willing to be vulnerable. When we are able to be vulnerable, we can admit that our own perceptions are merely that: our perceptions. Others see the same data we see, and they may see it differently. Often even our perceptions of our own actions are muddied by the fact that we're too close to them. Reflection gets all of our perceptions out into the open so that we can learn from them. Reflection helps us move from information to knowledge, from knowledge to understanding, and in those breakthrough moments, from understanding to wisdom.

Reflection Practices for Individuals

When we're aware of what we're thinking, what we're feeling, what triggers us, and what supports our ability to cope, we will make more mindful and proactive decisions. Without the sort of reflection that allows for self-knowledge, we may lose our sense of self. These are the times when we find ourselves feeling as though we're being dragged through our lives. With self-knowledge, and the sense of inner connection that comes with it, we will likely feel less victimized by our circumstances and more able to walk through the chaos calmly and effectively.

In this section we offer a variety of practical ways for individuals to cultivate mindfulness through self-reflection practices. Clearly our needs and preferences are unique to each of us, so not all of these particular practices may fit you. The important thing is to determine what does aid in your ability to cultivate mindfulness and self-knowing, and to commit to at least one or two practices that will help you participate more purposefully in your work and in your life.

Start Your Work with Intention

Setting your intention for the day can become a treasured way to care for yourself and prepare for the work you are called to do. It may be a time to remember that you are enough, exactly as you are. It may be a time to reflect on the knowledge that your capacity to convey compassion to others depends on the extent to which you have compassion for yourself. Consider the following possibilities for starting your day with intention:

- Spend time each morning in prayer.

- Practice seated meditation or walking meditation.

- Ritualize the time spent with your morning cup of coffee or tea, and round out that experience by reading a favorite passage or listening to an audio meditation.

- Intentionally use the commute to work as a time for quieting your mind.

- Use your entry into work as a time to notice something of beauty or meaning, and mindfully breathe it in as you walk from the parking lot to your office or work station.

- As soon as you arrive at work, pause and breathe deeply, and silently acknowledge and appreciate the beginning of a new day.

Reconnect With Your Purpose throughout Your Day

Remember why you are doing this important work. Some people find that carrying a symbol that has meaning for them in their pocket helps them remember their purpose during stressful times. Examples of symbols include a card with a message inscribed on it, a small stone with a meaningful word on it such as *breathe* or *compassion* or *grace* or *peace,* or some other personal token. This remembering can occur in a few moments of quiet contemplation by repeating a mantra that has meaning to you, through listening to a favorite meditation, or through a brief exchange with a trusted colleague. This remembering is not a one-time event, but rather an ongoing practice that helps you stay centered and clear about what you are called to do, who you intend to be, and why you're choosing to be part of any of it.

Intentionally Cultivate Mindfulness throughout Your Day

The idea that we can integrate mindful practices into our everyday lives is freeing. Without adding any more minutes to our day, we can develop ways to pause and be mindful in the moment. Remember the teaching of Thich Nhat Hanh (1992), who guides us to be aware of routine cues in our lives and to use them as "calls to mindfulness." Any of these events might work as such cues in a health care setting:

- a ringing phone

- a call bell

- the action of picking up the next chart

- the action of entering and leaving the unit

- the action of entering and leaving a patient's room

- the act of washing our hands

We can train ourselves to take any of these as cues to notice our breath and to breathe more mindfully. The cue may remind us to stand straighter, to relax our shoulders, to slow our pace, and to notice our energy.

Appreciate the Unexpected

We all know intellectually that caring for people is unpredictable and that the unexpected is the norm in health care. Yet when we are being truly honest with ourselves, most health care professionals admit that we like to control our worlds even though we know such control is an illusion. There is a wide variance in our individual capacities to "go with the flow" and cope gracefully with unexpected stressors. How we shape our own experience of the unexpected is our choice. We can appreciate it as something exciting—something that changes the direction of the energy around us and challenges us intellectually—or we can see it as a burden. The point is this: The unexpected is going to continue to happen whether we appreciate it or not, so if we make a reflective practice out of it we can move from merely tolerating the unexpected to allowing it to help us feel more vital and energized within our sometimes highly routinized work.

A beginning practice is to consciously expect the unexpected.

- Notice how you respond when you are faced with the unexpected.

- Notice the way you think about it, how your body responds, and what you experience emotionally.

- Do your thoughts serve your capacity to cope and respond effectively?

- What facilitates your ability to cope and what hinders it?

- Are you someone who inspires others to focus and come together with purpose during unexpected events?

Practice Time-shifting

While we can't slow down the people in our environment, we can be aware of our own pace and intentionally "time-shift" (Rechtschaffen, 1996) in order to slow down and to better match the needs of the patients and families in our care. Unless they consciously time-shift to a slower, calmer pace, many clinicians become entrained to an accelerated pace and lose the ability to attune to the people around them. Rechtschaffen echoes Thich Nhat Hanh's perspective on cultivating mindfulness using cues from everyday life, specifically his suggested practice of noticing the ordinary and honoring the mundane. The practice here is to begin consciously noticing your relationship with time. Here are some things to reflect on as you learn more about your relationship with time:

- Notice the ways in which you accelerate and decelerate your pace and whether your change in pace is based on actual needs or if you're simply more inclined to be entrained to the rhythm of those around you.

- Use the cue of hand washing to slow yourself down and reclaim your own rhythm. What other everyday cues would be effective in your work world?

- What are some ways you can take time to literally step out of the fast pace of your environment? Is it possible to use meal breaks, coffee breaks, or time spent laughing with a friend as opportunities for time-shifting?

- Find a place where you're able to walk slowly, quietly, and mindfully. Use this practice to cleanse yourself of the fast-paced rhythm of your work environment and shift your pace back to one that you consciously choose.

Transition with Intention

Many yoga classes end with a pose called Savasana. It's typically done lying down and it's a moment in which participants simultaneously release and integrate all of the energies taken in during the class. This is an apt metaphor for the end of a work period in health care, because it isn't the case that we want to simply forget all of the things we experience in our work. Since we work with and attune to human beings, we accumulate a lot of energies to assimilate, and assimilating those energies consciously can make for a more peaceful transition from work to home.

End your work period with intentional practices that allow you to integrate both the highs and lows. There are activities that can help us to mindfully release whatever stresses we've taken on and to prepare ourselves to engage in relationship with others outside of work. This can be the mindful use of cues that would give us a sense of closure—a closing prayer, or washing our hands and releasing the stresses of our day down the drain. It could be the practice of consistently offering a word of encouragement to those who are taking over where we left off.

Additionally, saying goodbye to each of the patients in our care creates a more comfortable transitional experience for them and for us. Just as tending to the beginning, middle, and end of each therapeutic encounter is part of the holding of patients, we hold ourselves when we acknowledge the beginnings, middles, and endings in our own experience. Clinicians tell us often that when they go home they don't have anything left to give, and they worry that those they love the most get the least of them.

Clinicians tell us often that when they go home they don't have anything left to give, and they worry that those they love the most get the least of them.

Transitioning with intention helps us to refuel as we move into the next phase of our lives.

- What has worked for you in the past to transition gracefully from work to the rest of your life? Is there a practice that worked for you at one time but is now no longer your habit?

- What are some practices or rituals you could try to help you transition more intentionally from work to home?

- What might help you enter your home and connect with those you love with intention, positive energy, and a peaceful heart?

You can choose to use your walk out of work as a time in which you intentionally ask yourself what you most appreciated about the work time, your patients, your colleagues, or yourself. On your walk out, you can make it a practice to ask yourself questions such as these:

- What did I learn today?

- To whom did I feel most connected today and why?

- What am I most grateful for today?

Find a Reflection Partner

Some people are willing and able to engage in reflection completely on their own. They may enjoy journaling, art, walking meditation, or guided meditation through reading or listening to audio recordings. But others need the chance to process our thoughts and emotions out loud with someone we respect and trust. In seeking out a reflection partner, look for someone you can go to in moments of intensity when your mind is clouded or when you are feeling distressed. When your practices seem to be failing and your ability to process on your own isn't giving you clarity, have someone selected in advance to whom you can go. If you decide that you'd benefit from having a reflective partner, there are some things to consider as you seek out and nurture this important professional relationship.

Choose Someone with Whom You Feel Completely Safe

"I need two minutes to process with you about why I'm having such a hard time with Mrs. T." It's important to cultivate a relationship in which you feel safe to be vulnerable about anything that's challenging you. You must also feel secure that this person will respect and care for you by keeping your conversations confidential. If you have any doubts about the integrity of a potential reflection partner, keep looking.

Choose Someone Whose Opinion and Counsel You Trust

Choose a person who is committed to your growth. It may be that the best choice for a reflection partner is not your closest work friend. You're not looking for someone to validate you in your grievances, but rather for someone who will challenge you and say, "This has come up for you three times; let's look at what part in this is yours to own." This can be a peer relationship, or you may also choose to foster a reflection partnership with someone you see more as a mentor or coach. In a mentor-mentee relationship, the reflection is not necessarily mutual; it's more guided and the agreement is that this mentor, whom you trust for his or her emotional intelligence and/or years of experience, will help you grow in the way that you want to grow.

Your reflection partner could be a person who is available to talk with you in person, or it can be a relationship in which you communicate through email correspondence or telephone conversations. While conversing in person may seem preferable, we have found that a variety of approaches can work. For example, an email journal shared with a colleague provides a written record so that you can reflect on your reflection. Email or telephone conversations can be extraordinarily convenient as they can happen at unusual times outside the work setting. The key is having sanctioned time and a go-to person for the purpose of reflecting to gain greater clarity, wisdom, and peace in your practice.

Practical Reflection Methods for Groups

There are many reasons to expand a personal practice of reflection to include reflection with a group of peers. Reflection facilitates learning for groups as much as it does for individuals, and it also provides us with an opportunity to gather with our peers in a less hurried, less stressful, more focused environment. As we gather for group reflection, we learn things about each other that may never have surfaced during our usual professional interactions, and as this information is shared new bonds are created. Even if the subject of the group reflection has nothing to do with building teamwork, the very act of spending time together in a formalized way—out of the normal work environment, tapping into our collective wisdom—builds collegiality among team members. As we've said several times, everyone has a back story, and reflection often brings the elements of people's back story forward. As we learn more about our peers and discover things about ourselves with our peers as compassionate witnesses, a deeper sense of connection blooms.

Before we discuss examples of group reflection practices, we want to introduce two bodies of knowledge that we believe are foundational for group reflective practice. They are circle practice and Appreciative Inquiry.

Circle Practice

Circle practice helps us slow down and focus on the subject we've gathered to discuss. Meeting in a circle is an ancient human tradition. Circle practice is a form of meeting in which people have gathered together, often around a fire, for respectful communication, to learn about each other, to share stories, and to make decisions about matters of importance. Margaret Wheatley (2010), a writer and leadership consultant who studies organizational behavior, says this:

It is important to remember this long, loving lineage as we now daily sit in rows in classrooms, auditoriums, buses, and airplanes looking at the back of each other's head . . . After all these centuries of separation and isolation, circle welcomes us back into a shape where we can listen, be heard, and be respected, where we can think and create together. (p. ix)

PeerSpirit, Inc. is an educational company founded in 1994 by Christina Baldwin and Ann Linnea with a mission to teach circle practice to groups of people around the world who are devoted to learning through reflection and meaningful conversation (www.peerspirit.com). Circle practice offers a structure and methodology to create an "interpersonal net" formed by the shared intentions and commitment of the members of the reflection group (Baldwin, 1998). Baldwin and Linnea say that there is something about the formation of a circle that "turns people into participatory learners and leaders" (2010, p. xv). The circle structure and methodology facilitate safety and respectful connection between participants, and this accelerates honest exchange and collective discovery. There are three valuable assumptions that support circle practice (Baldwin & Linnea, 2010):

- The wisdom we need is in the room.

- Every voice matters and contributes to the greater good.

- Slowing down, reflecting, and talking together can help us be more effective and productive.

The structure, principles, and practices of circle create a safe container for reflection and learning. The center of the circle symbolizes the reason or purpose for the gathering. Remembering that the ancient roots of circle began with the fire in the center, the center in circle practice holds the symbolic fire around which the participants gather. For this reason, the center should hold something of meaning for the group. Examples of meaningful symbols include a mission or purpose statement, a statement of commitment to patients and families, a symbol to represent a therapeutic concept that the group wants to focus on, flowers to represent growth and beauty, a candle to represent healing, or any other symbol that has meaning and purpose for the group.

Remembering that the ancient roots of circle began with the fire in the center, the center in circle practice holds the symbolic fire around which the participants gather.

Three basic practices guide the interaction of the participants in the circle:

1. The first practice is listening with attention. Listening is the contribution we make to one another in circle. Attentive listening is the practice of giving the one speaking your undivided attention.

2. The second practice is speaking with intention. It requires us to be self-aware and to focus our stories, knowledge, information, and inquiry on the purpose or topic of the circle.

3. The third practice is tending to the well-being of the whole group. This means that each individual remains aware of the impact of his or her contribution on the others in the group.

Baldwin and Linnea propose that in order to support our ability to be aware of our contributions in circle, we ask ourselves questions such as these (2010, p. 28):

- What is my motivation or hope for sharing this particular thought or comment?

- How do I offer my contribution in a way that will benefit what we're doing?

- How will I consider what I say before I say it and still speak my "truth?"

The circle serves as a practice field for being in healthy and respectful relationships. The attention to the emotional safety of participants occurs through forming agreements between members, interacting with unconditional respect for each individual, listening, and seeing each person as a human being who matters. It's important that time is spent in creating the circle as a safe container for group members to get to know, appreciate, and trust each other. The practices facilitate connection and trust among participants which help to create the space for learning. When we engage in circle practice over time, it gets inside of us. Circle participants report being able to remember and access the quiet wisdom of the circle as they go about their daily lives. The personal awareness and respectful interaction that occur in circle practice become a way of being.

Appreciative Inquiry (AI)

Appreciative Inquiry (AI) is a philosophy and methodology for discovering and growing the best in each of us. It originated as a model of change leadership at Case Western Reserve University's School of Management in 1980 (Cooperrider & Whitney, 2005). While AI is typically used as a methodology to promote system-wide organizational transformation, its principles can be used very effectively in reflective practice for groups or for individuals.

Appreciative Inquiry offers a "strength-based" approach that guides us to build on what is working by reflecting on stories of success, rather than correcting what isn't working. Some may think that this mindset is too idealistic—that it is not rooted in the real world of obstacles, problems, and failures. But experience shows that AI does not ignore reality. Instead, the methodology harnesses the already forward-moving energy of those in the culture who are striving for excellence. A senior executive described his experience with AI in the following excerpt from Cooperrider and Whitney (2005):

> *Appreciative Inquiry can get you much better results than seeking out and solving problems. That's an interesting concept for me—because [we] are among the best problem solvers in the world. We troubleshoot everything. . . . We concentrate enormous resources on correcting problems that have relatively minor impact on overall service and performance . . . this approach can create a negative culture. If you combine a negative culture with all the challenges we face today, it could be easy to convince ourselves that we have too many problems to overcome—to slip into a paralyzing sense of hopelessness. Don't get me wrong. I'm not advocating mindless happy talk. AI is a complex science designed to make things better. We can't ignore problems—we just need to approach them from the other side. (p. 5)*

AI is built on the premise that the wisdom is within us and that it's in learning to ask the right kinds of questions that we can begin to uncover that wisdom. It's a way to discover insights and possibilities that we couldn't discover otherwise. AI suggests that if something is already happening, it can almost assuredly happen more often and could potentially become a systemic reality.

A psychological phenomenon occurs when we look at what we *can* do instead of what we can't do. People become involved and energetic. Possibilities, ideas, and creativity flourish.

The construction of the questions themselves is extremely important, as they directly influence how the group will respond. Powerful, relevant questions accelerate exploration and discovery. According to AI methodology, questions are seen as more powerful if they influence group engagement and inspire exploration, and they are seen as less powerful if they elicit a "yes or no" response. While the construction of good questions is an art form that is beyond the scope of this book, we recommend the book, *The Art of Powerful Questions: Catalyzing Insight, Innovation, and Action* (2003) by Eric Vogt, David Isaacs, and Juanita Brown as a resource. Some examples of appreciative questions that promote reflection and deepen our knowledge and understanding are included here as models for you to build on:

- Describe a time when you have been face to face with a patient's anger and you successfully defused the situation or brought comfort to the person expressing anger. What challenged you? What surprised you?

- Think of a colleague who is consistently present and attuned and able to manage conflicting demands most of the time. Describe what you see and experience. What contributes to her capacity to manage so effectively? What do you notice and most appreciate about what she is doing? What do you notice and appreciate about what she is not doing?

- When has the act of wondering with a patient or on a patient's behalf led to a positive outcome? What facilitates your ability to wonder? What are some ways we can support the practice of wondering with our patients and with each other?

- What has been your most memorable experience of holding a patient or patient's family member? When have you felt held by a colleague or your entire team? What are some ways you hold colleagues in your practice? What challenges you? What inspires you?

Examples of Reflection Groups

We've gathered several examples of group reflection practices that we know are going on in organizations and communities across the country. Some may be familiar to you. In fact they may already be alive and thriving in your organization. Others may show you new opportunities for development. The implementation of some of these practices will require broader organizational involvement, and some of them can be done on a very small scale and simply require a group of committed practitioners.

Book Groups

Book groups are an effective method for helping health care professionals deepen their knowledge and understanding of people's experience of illness and care. This book has been written to serve this purpose, and many other books lend themselves beautifully to group reflection and study. There are compelling books written by people who have experienced life-changing trauma and acute or chronic illness. Through their descriptive writing we are invited into the mind and heart of the person actually living with and coping with the illness experience. When we take in their experience through reading and reflection, we deepen our knowledge, understanding, and wisdom, and thereby become more attuned to the meaning and magnitude of the illness experience to the person and their loved ones in our care. Here are three excellent books for group reflection in a health care setting:

I'm Here: Compassionate Communication in Patient Care (2010), by Marcus Engel

Marcus Engel writes that while modern medical technology helps patients recover faster than in any other time in history, the human interaction between patient and caregiver is still the essential foundation of healing. *I'm Here* is a personal narrative from the patient's perspective. After being blinded and suffering catastrophic injuries at the hands of a drunk driver, Marcus Engel endured years of hospitalization, rehab, and recovery. He teaches us about profound vulnerability, loss, and the capacity we have as humans to heal and make a difference in our world. This book is filled with practical advice, irreverence, and humor as well as great appreciation for all who are called to care.

My Stroke of Insight: A Brain Scientist's Personal Journey (2006), by Jill Bolte Taylor

At the age of 37, Jill Bolte Taylor, a neuroanatomist at Harvard, suffered a burst blood vessel in the left side of her brain. Her knowledge of the anatomy and function of the brain allowed her to observe and understand her rapid loss of mental capacity as well as what it took to regain her health and ability to contribute as a scientist once again—a journey that took eight years. In Bolte Taylor's terms, she needed to be "rebuilt," learning to read, to dress herself, to drive a car, and to think. During this time she explored her right brain's natural capacity for achieving wisdom and peace. She writes, "My stroke of insight is that at the core of my right hemisphere consciousness is a character that is directly connected to my feelings of deep inner peace" (p. 133). Bolte Taylor writes eloquently about her feelings when caregivers were attuned and present—the precious moments in which she felt a "safe" energy around her— as well as about those times when caregivers were not attuned and made her feel afraid and vulnerable.

Beyond Rage: The Emotional Impact of Chronic Physical Illness (1985), by JoAnn LeMaistre

We came upon this book in our quest to understand the dynamics of chronic illness as our daughter courageously copes with it every day. JoAnn LeMaistre says that most chronic illness sufferers feel alone and isolated when they have little understanding of the natural stages of emotional response to chronic physical illness. Learning about these patterns of emotional response can help people live a higher quality of life despite their physical challenges. She says that physicians and other health care professionals tend to focus on the physical symptoms and sometimes neglect the critical emotional factors. We have also heard from clinicians that they struggle with some of the responses and behaviors of people suffering from chronic illness. We think we can all benefit from greater understanding of the impact that critical illness has on patients, families, and caregivers alike and of the emotional patterns often seen in such patients and their families. JoAnn LeMaistre is a clinical psychologist who counsels the chronically ill and their families. She has multiple sclerosis and her sight and muscular capabilities have been seriously compromised. She is an inspiring example of living fully and "able-hearted" with chronic illness.

Facilitated Narrative Exchange and Reflective Practice

Facilitated Narrative Exchange and Reflective Practice is the terminology used to describe a reflective process that was implemented and evaluated by Lorraine Dickey and her colleagues (2011) at Lehigh Valley Hospital and Health Network. This approach to reflective practice was used to educate staff in reflection in order to promote cultural changes needed to successfully implement and integrate Patient and Family-Centered Care philosophies in the NICU and pediatric units.

To address the cultural and professional barriers, Dickey et al. implemented and evaluated a facilitated small-group narrative exchange and reflective practice model based on Rita Charon's work in narrative medicine (Charon, 2006).

The method described by Dickey and colleagues proceeded as follows:

1. Open discussions were held with pediatric and NICU nursing staff members and physicians to identify why they felt it was difficult to support patient and family-centered care on a 24/7 basis.

2. In collaboration with the hospital ethnographer the facilitator team developed a voluntary participant survey with both qualitative and quantitative components to evaluate the effectiveness of the two reflective practice initiatives.

3. Their primary goal was to develop self-and other-awareness and insights through reflective writing and narrative exchange.

Dickey and her colleagues conclude that narrative reflection is a promising method for improving "clinical care and the lived experiences of the professionals" (p 132). Additionally, they see great promise for using narrative reflection to facilitate "interdisciplinary agreement about patient safety, medical errors, and collaboration on questions of retention, attrition, and interprofessional relations" (p. 132). We also see great promise for enhancing interdisciplinary knowledge and understanding of patients' and families' emotional response to illness and crisis.

Patient Observation

Patient observation is practiced at St. Luke's Methodist Hospital in Cedar Rapids, Iowa, according to Chief Clinical Officer, Mary Ann Osborn (personal communication, January 27, 2012). The purpose of the patient observation is to gain greater understanding of the care experience through the eyes of the patient and family. A clinician is assigned to be in a patient's room for approximately 45 minutes while other clinicians carry out their usual interactions and responsibilities. Permission for the observation is granted by the patients being observed or by the patients' families.

After the observation, there is a debriefing between the observing clinician and a representative of the observation program. The results of the debriefing are then brought to a larger committee which reflects on the cumulative findings and makes recommendations for changes. The work of this committee has been very practically focused—for example, identifying possible patient irritants such as extraneous noise in the environment and the temperature of the room. They have also begun to identify duplicative and inefficient practices. We see a strong potential for these sorts of observations to be used as a way to deepen learning and understanding of the therapeutic practices as well. The debriefing session includes reflective questions like these:

- What, if anything, did the clinician do that indicated that he or she saw the patient as a person?

- Describe the caregiver's use of touch.

- What did you notice about how the clinician spoke (or didn't speak) to the patient?

- What did you notice about the way caregivers were attuned to the patient and family?

- What specific examples of the clinician's behavior reflect wondering, following, and/or holding?

Schwartz Rounds

Schwartz Rounds are scheduled meetings of caregivers from all disciplines and specialties who meet to discuss the relational aspects of practice. Founded in memory of Kenneth Schwartz shortly after his death in 1995 from lung cancer, and set up according to his final wishes, these rounds address the universal need for caregivers to talk about what it's like to deal with the difficult emotional and social issues we face every day. Schwartz Rounds are specifically designed to help practitioners integrate what they've learned in their relational practice, particularly what Schön calls the "swampy lowlands" of clinical practice (1987), in which answers are often anything but clear. One participant put it this way: "Rounds are a place where people who don't usually talk about the heart of the work are willing to share their vulnerability, to question themselves. Rounds are an opportunity for dialogue that doesn't happen anywhere else in the hospital." Schwartz Rounds include patients as well as caregivers.

Schwartz Rounds are now regular occurrences in 240 health care facilities in 35 states (The Schwartz Center, 2011). These organizations provide regularly scheduled meetings that health care professionals can count on as their time to reflect on their own experiences, learn from the experiences of others, and integrate all of their learning, deepening their wisdom along the way.

Patients and families who participate in Schwartz Rounds view the organizations that sponsor them as compassionate, caring facilities. They understand how important it must be to the people in the organization to give great care, since those caregivers actually want to learn from patients and families.

The process of telling their stories is inspiring to patients because they see how their own suffering can benefit others. Having the group bear witness to their suffering is a healing experience for them.

Nursing Salons

Founded by Marie Manthey in 2001, nursing salons provide nurses in all stages of their careers the chance to reflect together on their work. Manthey began holding salons in her home to provide nurses with a place to engage in dialogue about the challenges and triumphs they're experiencing in their work. The evenings feature "talk that amuses, challenges, and amazes and is sometimes passionately acted upon" (2007). Although most attendees are nurses, anyone with a desire to enter into conversation about nursing practice is welcome. The monthly salons include a meal, as breaking bread together is another way to "create the circle," and the fact that everything is provided for participants removes some potential barriers to attending.

Manthey's salons have grown over the years. The most frequent comments on her blog acknowledge the great relief participants feel that in this time in which so many clinicians work in a negative atmosphere and under high stress, the salons are consistently positive and grounding, enabling participants to explore the ways in which they are inherently empowered in the clinician-patient relationships they create. Nursing salons are now being held throughout the country as well as in the UK. They're all voluntary and are driven by a shared passion to reflect, grow, and support each other.

In your own professional environment, the salon concept could easily be expanded to include an interdisciplinary group to talk about how best to provide compassionate patient care or about how to overcome the challenges in our work. Salons could be held monthly throughout the year, off site, and begin with a check-in round followed by a simple question such as, "What is on your mind about . . . (your practice, etc.)?" The ground rules for a salon are the same as for any other reflection group: participants agree to maintain confidentiality and to hold each attendee in love and esteem. At the end of the salon, there is a check-out in which individuals talk about what new awareness they're taking with them into their lives and their practice.

Manthey's nursing salons begin and end with the same question: "What is on your mind about nursing?" The use of the same question for check-in and check-out helps the group to measure its progress. Manthey says of her salons that "the function is healing and the outcome is hope" (Manthey, 2010).

> *Novice nurses feel hope when they realize that seasoned staff nurses are still as passionate about nursing practice as they are. Veteran nurses feel the same hope as they see new nurses' depth of caring and passion about nursing. It becomes so clear to everyone that nursing is a culture, not just a job. (p. 19)*

Re-Igniting the Spirit of Caring

Re-Igniting the Spirit of Caring is a three-day reflective workshop for all members of health care organizations (Koloroutis, 2011). It incorporates circle practice and Appreciative Inquiry as participants are invited to reconnect with the power and purpose of their work. The curriculum is framed around the three critical relationships for the provision of humane and compassionate care: relationship with self, relationship with colleagues, and relationship with patients and their families. The participants' learning and interactions are guided by these questions:

- Who am I as a person and as a caregiver?

- What do I need to know about myself to support my work and care of others?

- What can I do to maximize my energy for my work and also have energy for my personal life?

- How do I find and sustain joy, meaning, and purpose in my work and life?

- What do I contribute and what do I need in order to create healthy relationships with my colleagues?

- What does it mean in my work and within our organization to provide world-class care for patients and families?

- Does my work matter? How do I know I am making a meaningful difference?

The three-day retreat provides participants with time to step away from the stress and chaos of the health care setting and engage in reflection and dialogue. This sanctioned time creates a safe container and a "practice field" for experiencing respectful and intentional relationships with each other and with the patients and families who join the health care participants on the second day of the retreat. Each patient or family guest briefly shares his or her story about needing and receiving care and then participates in a small group reflection and dialogue with the health care participants on which parts of their experience were caring and which were not.

Integrating Reflection into Existing Group Processes

Reflection doesn't necessarily have to take a great deal of extra time since much of our already-scheduled time together as groups and teams can provide us with opportunities for reflection. Huddles and scheduled staff meetings can include time for team reflection. While more time might be spent formally "creating the circle" in groups that meet outside of work, there are efficient ways to mark the beginning and end of any group's time together that can be very effective in focusing and creating a sense of common purpose within the group. If huddles and scheduled staff meetings follow circle practice to even a small extent, participants are more likely to feel connected and therefore more willing to engage in the kind of vulnerability that makes reflection effective.

Huddles

Huddles can be used to formalize being mindful as a team. Team huddles are prominent right now in many health care settings. To maximize the use of the valuable time together, a team could use huddles not only to plan logistics together but also to be mindful about the meaning and purpose of the work. To create the circle in this setting, it's helpful to mark the beginning of the meeting formally by the ringing of a chime, a brief reading, a patient story of appreciation, or simply a moment of silence and breathing together. Some faith-based organizations start meetings with prayer. These practices help the group begin its work mindfully and from a point of common purpose and commitment. Formalizing this practice helps people remember to let go of grudges or issues from the past, to affirm that we all have each other's back, to review the agreements to which we have committed as a team, and to help us focus on seeing and attuning to the people in our care. Ending the team huddle time with a formalized practice also helps the group to settle its energy before beginning the shift.

Huddles are a great time to remind team members of the moments in which they can choose to be especially mindful.

Huddles are a great time to remind team members of the moments in which they can choose to be especially mindful. For example, a hand-off between one clinician and another can work as a cue for remembering purpose as well as reflecting on the meaning of this transition to the patient. Remembering to say hello to patients and team members at the beginning of a shift and goodbye at the end of one can help us to hold our patients and colleagues.

Scheduled Staff Meetings

Staff meetings have a potential for connection that is often overlooked. The biggest problem with scheduled staff meetings is that people are often too pulled back into their work to be fully present (or even physically present) for the duration of the meeting. Many people spend that time looking at their text messages or dashing out of the room to take care of patients. We know that it will be hard for some readers to imagine bringing an element of calm reflection to meetings such as these. To make the most of these meetings, create time in which some people are covering the care of the patients so that others may attend the meeting with focus.

Historically, staff meetings are primarily information-driven and problem-focused, but what would it take for reflection to be integrated as a core part of the agenda? What would it take to reorganize the way information is provided so that reflection and dialogue comprise a higher percentage of the content of each meeting? This reflection could be appreciative in nature, such as:

- What are you most proud of in your practice over the past week or so?

- What was your experience with the therapeutic practices of wondering, following, and holding this week?

- What one thing have you learned this week that would help in your therapeutic care of patients and their families?

- What are some ways in which you have visibly demonstrated that you have the backs of your team members?

- What is one successful practice you have used this week to take care of yourself?

A byproduct of this kind of reflective practice is that team members make more visible how they're thinking about their practice, which results in greater collective learning, vulnerability, compassion, and team support. In order for this time to be used effectively for reflection, it's essential that time and focus be given to creating a sense of trust and safety within the group. It helps for the group to agree on some ground rules for how people will interact during this time so that people feel safe talking openly about their practice. These meetings are not the time to air grievances or to mediate disagreements. The culture of the group will develop over time, and it's important that it be guided by the principles of mutual respect, trust, open and honest communication, and consistent and visible support.

The research of scientists and learning theorists such as Daniel Siegel, Chris Argyris, Russell Ackoff, and Donald Schön tells us that reflection is fundamental to integrating learning. Reflection is what turns otherwise meaningless data into something that we can use to enrich our lives and the lives of those around us. According to Siegel (2006), who refers to reflection as the "fourth 'R'" of education, reflection helps us integrate and "rewire" the prefrontal cortex of our brains, thus cultivating a greater capacity for being mindful and present. The work of Siegel,

Reflection is what turns otherwise meaningless data into something that we can use to enrich our lives and the lives of those around us.

Argyris, Ackoff, and Schön supports a shift in our thinking so that reflection is viewed not as a luxury but rather as a mainstream component of professional education and development. What would it take for us to balance our resources so that we can invest in reflective learning in the same way we currently invest in technical education? What would it take for us to balance our investment in learning both the relational and instrumental elements of our patient care so that we can truly achieve extraordinary results?

Reflections on the Therapeutic Relationship in Practice: Stories for Individual and Team Reflection

In this section we offer two stories and one meditation about therapeutic care that lend themselves to individual and team reflection. The first story, "Adam the Pharmacist," comes from our own experience. We thank Adrienne Hopkins for sharing the second story, "A Sturdy Presence." Michael wrote the meditation "So I Get Tired, and I Forget" for the *See Me As a Person* CD (Trout, 2011).These narratives may be useful for reflecting together to reinforce the therapeutic practices.

Adam the Pharmacist: Through the Eyes of a Family

He was tall and lanky, and his eyes were dancing before he even spoke. But there was really nothing about his appearance that would have given a clue that this man was about to transform our daughter's health care experience.

We were at a huge university medical complex, and we weren't there for the food. Alicia was being seen in the clinic for renal failure two years after her lupus was discovered. Her mother, Mary, was a match, and ultimately they both would be admitted—not only to different units, but to different hospitals within the complex—for a kidney transplant.

Adam, a pharmacist specializing in medicine for transplant patients, was going to be in and out a great deal over the next several days. (Little did we know then that he was going to be in and out of our lives many times in the coming years.) He would be our teacher and guide. After all, Alicia was going to become intimately familiar with the drugs he would bring, and she will remain so for the rest of her life. The list of side effects and cautions made our heads spin.

What was it about this guy? How did he know how to make a vulnerable but feisty 16-year-old feel comfortable and ready to take in the mountains of information he was about to impart? Why was he talking to our daughter about who she is, what she likes to do, and what her life is like? And why was she (obviously in no state of mind to be gregarious) responding cheerfully, telling him all about herself? She looked suddenly optimistic, and she was laughing for the first time in weeks.

Then, just a moment later, Adam shifted from informal conversation to teaching; it was seamless. How did he do that? He had boring minutiae to impart. It didn't matter, really, that this minutia was key to saving Alicia's life; it was still boring and it was too much for an irritable adolescent girl. So he pulled out flash cards! She said, with unexpected enthusiasm, "I love flash-cards." (She did?)

How is it that Alicia was for this man so much more than a name on a file, a diagnosis, a patient facing a serious medical procedure? From the moment he first walked into Alicia's room, this caregiver (because it was clear that he saw himself first and foremost as a giver of care) was open, curious, and full of wonder about the person he was about to discover. And a scared little girl, not known at the time for her gentleness and openness, opened right up and permitted her vulnerability to be seen.

By the end of their first encounter, Adam had taught Alicia the ins and outs of what would become her new drug regimen, but more importantly, he had begun to empower her.

Adam connected with who Alicia was. He asked questions, he listened, and they built a relationship together. Oddly, his small investment of time and authentic curiosity began reaping benefits right away. Not only did she listen, she retained, and in spite of how onerous the role of medications is in her life, years later she still manages them with humor and meticulousness. She made an investment in what this man was teaching. Because Adam took the time to make a connection and to lay the foundation for a relationship, pharmaceutical efficacy and adherence to the medication requirements soared. Our daughter's knowledge base expanded. Their encounter was always professional, never lacking in personal boundaries, but it was about more than just medication. It was about helping her to cope with illness, with surgery, with pain, with drug side-effects, and with the awful realization that she must commit to these drugs for the rest of her days.

Adam helped our little girl to believe in herself. And it was a first step in her believing that she would be able to manage her illness and to lead her own life.

Adam stayed connected with Alicia through other hospitalizations as well. As the pharmacist on the transplant team, his role was to see all transplant patients. His position was such that when he visited he always had some pharmacy responsibility to fulfill with her, but his ongoing relationship with her was consistently therapeutic in that Alicia-the-Person was always more important to him than anything else.

About four years after her transplant, Alicia was hospitalized with a threatened rejection of her kidney, and Adam showed up every day to reinforce—more through attentiveness and listening than through anything he said—that she was capable and important. In her college years, Alicia once had to go to the emergency room in the middle of the night while we were out of town. As Adam had given us his card and invited us to contact him if we ever needed help, we called him. He arrived at 6:00 the next morning to see her. She was later discharged from the ER for immediate admission to the hospital, but there was no bed on the transplant wing. She sat in the admitting area for almost eight hours waiting for a bed. Adam stopped in to see her several times throughout the day just to see how she was holding up. We found out later that he also made sure that the things that mattered most to Alicia (for example that she be treated as a young adult and not as a child, or that she was distressed at missing school and worried about how long she would be in the hospital) were shared with other members of the team. Every now and again someone would have knowledge of something important about Alicia-the-Person that could be traced back to Adam having shared it on her behalf.

Adam's whole interaction with Alicia, from beginning to end, looked effortless. His goals as a pharmacist were to help her learn how to manage her disease and to assure that she had the correct medication regime. His role as a caregiver was to connect with her as a person, and in so doing, he helped her to cope with her illness and begin to take charge of her life.

But most of all, he was there.

The story of Adam the Pharmacist is a portrait of a clinician that any individual or care team may find worth further reflection. What made this connection seem so effortless? What one thing might you take from this story to apply to your own practice?

The following story is quite different, though it is also a story of exemplary care. In this case, however, the masterful clinician offers more with his quiet presence than with his words.

A Sturdy Presence: Through the Eyes of a Patient's Daughter

I had always known that my father's alcoholism would steal away the years of his life. Still, as much as I tried to prepare myself, seeing him on life support stirred up a whirlwind of powerful emotions. Cirrhosis of the liver had advanced the deterioration of his condition so quickly. I knew my role that day would require me to be strong and stoic, but inside I felt like a small child. I wished he would reassure me that everything would be all right. I longed for him to comfort me.

I had accompanied my father to the hospital on numerous occasions. I'd felt and heard the judgments passed against him because of his alcoholism. He had been warned about the dangers of his drinking, yet here we were. I couldn't help but wonder what the staff would think. Would they feel that he deserved this fate? Would they see him only as a 59-year-old drunk? I wished they could have a glimpse into our past, with insight into the man who held me on his lap and read me the same book every night with fresh excitement because he knew it was my favorite; the man who worked hard and went without so that his family was taken care of; the man who played his harmonica and sang; the man who loved life and loved his children. Would they recognize that man behind all the tubes, IVs, and complicated equipment? Would they recognize the person behind his diagnosis? It mattered to me that he was allowed to die with dignity.

When I entered the room, my fears were alleviated. These people were clearly able to see the man behind the diagnosis.

As he continued to decline, eventually it was time to unhook the respirator. Even though I knew that this was what he wanted, I was feeling very anxious. My father's nurse could see my discomfort and he asked to speak with me. He spent some time preparing me for what it would be like when my father passed—particularly that he might gasp for air, which can be very difficult to watch. He promised me that he would keep my father pain-free.

He also promised that he would be there through the entire experience, and he encouraged my family to take a few moments to do what we needed to do to tell my father good-bye.

Once they removed the respirator, we had the gift of 40 minutes with my father. His eyes were open and he was alert as my sister and I told stories and reassured him that it was his time to go and that we would take care of each other. There is one moment in particular that will always be with me. My father made a loud gurgle followed by a gasp. My sister screamed and ran to the foot of the bed. My stomach tightened with panic as I squeezed my father's hand. At that point I looked up and saw my father's nurse in the corner of the room. His eyes comforted me. He was a sturdy presence, off in the far corner, like an angel. I took comfort in the fact that he was standing like a sentry, ready to do anything to protect us but still allowing the experience to be 100% ours.

After my father transitioned, I thanked the nurse for his support. Because of his presence, a potentially scary experience was transformed into a beautiful gift. His guidance allowed me to be fully present with my father in the final moments of his journey.

So far we've reflected on the experiences of two patients being held in the care of exemplary clinicians. While the caregivers in these stories seem tireless in their care, we know that the intensity of most health care environments makes it almost impossible for us to bring our most focused, most professional self to each encounter every time. Here is a meditation that chronicles the very real experience of what it's like to question whether we have what it takes to keep going in those moments when it all seems like too much.

So I Get Tired, and I Forget

OK, so I get tired.
Real tired, some days.
Wiped right out, to tell you the truth.

And in such states,
I'm prone to forget why I'm doing this.
And so, some days, I forget how to do it.

It happens most when the limits of my power
are shoved quite in my face.
I see that I can't make this patient get better.
I can't make this patient be nice to me.
I can't even make my colleagues be nice to me.
I keep pouring energy into this work,
these people,
this place,
and it seems to drain out a hole somewhere.

These are important times for me.
When such times don't bring me completely to my knees,
they help me to reorganize myself,
to re-think the whole proposition,
to re-establish my priorities,
and to commit
once more
to the few things I can do:
To look after my next patient with compassion.
To breathe.
To remember that I am enough,
as I pour into each vessel what I can.
To be ready for the slightest hint of improvement,
or a moment when someone is grateful,
while not actually counting on it.
And to not be too shocked when neither this hospital

nor this patient
nor anybody else
stands up and salutes.
Let me today be a witness.
Let me give up rights to the outcome.
Let me suit up.
Let me show up.
Let me be the carrier of hope
for those who have little of their own.
But, mostly, let me just be there.

Summary of Key Thoughts

- We seem to be built with both the need to reflect on the important things in our lives and the facility to do just that. Under less hurried circumstances, we would naturally do reflection.

- We don't just do. We do, we notice our doing, we consider what we did, and we integrate and learn from what we did, so that our next doing is informed by past doing. All the while, we think about the context of our doing, and we modify our doing in response to that context.

- We are obligated to reflect on ourselves, on our patients, and on our work each day as if such reflection were as important as the acts we are reflecting upon—which, as it turns out, it is.

- Reflection is what transforms wondering, following, and holding from a way of thinking and a way of acting into a way of being.

- If the goal is to have permanent access to the wisdom we recognize as valuable, we have to put time and intention into applying it in our lives and reflecting on what we're learning.

- The instrumental aspects of our practice are highly conducive to algorithms and protocols and are frequently taught and learned through lecture, application, and observation in practice. The relational aspects of care are less black and white.

- Reflection helps us to notice and address those elements of our practice that defy predictability and technique.

- Though reflection doesn't necessarily produce perfect answers, it may produce novel perspectives, an alternative idea, or a new way to approach a situation in which nothing else has been working.

- A key factor in our ability to reflect is whether we have learned to embrace our own emotional vulnerability.

- Reflection challenges us to move beyond our most comfortable conclusions. It requires a vulnerability that allows us to risk being wrong, to operate without the net of scientific certainty, and to walk into a room with intelligent ignorance.

- According to Chris Argyris, highly educated people tend to perceive that they have a professional responsibility to "already know" and that their job is to offer their skills and intelligence. Embarrassment about not knowing enough or not being good enough is a barrier that these high achievers experience to reflecting on their own performance.

- The kind of vulnerability necessary for reflection celebrates our ability to admit that we may have something new to learn, and that our wisdom comes from not thinking we have to know it all.

- There is great value in looking at a situation in which something has worked unexpectedly.

- Reflection with a group facilitates access to "collective intelligence" which helps us move from information to knowledge, from knowledge to understanding, and in those breakthrough moments, from understanding to wisdom.

- With self-knowledge and the sense of inner connection that comes with it, we will likely feel less victimized by our circumstances and more able to "walk through the chaos" calmly and effectively.

- Everyone has a back story, and reflection often brings the elements of people's back story forward. As we learn more about our peers (and perhaps discover things about ourselves with our peers as our compassionate witnesses), a deeper sense of connection blooms.

- There is something about the formation of a circle that "turns people into participatory learners and leaders."

- The circle structure and methodology facilitate safety and respectful connection between participants that accelerate honest exchange and collective discovery.

- Appreciative Inquiry (AI) offers a "strength-based" approach that guides us to build on what is working by reflecting on stories of success rather than correcting what isn't working.

- Models of group reflection include book groups, narrative reflection sessions and workshops, patient observations, Schwartz Rounds, nursing salons, and Re-Igniting the Spirit of Caring workshops.

- Huddles and scheduled staff meetings can include time for team reflection.

Reflection

- Consider this statement: "I run out of the hospital and I run into the car and I run home and I am met with three children who all want my attention." How might an intentional transition help this caregiver refuel mentally, physically, and emotionally before returning home?

- What triggers you in caring for patients? What tends to offend you? If you become offended by something you hear, do you put up your defenses or do you become more curious, wondering about why you were so triggered? In what ways are you being served by shutting down? In what ways are you being served by becoming more curious?

- What reflective practices in this chapter appeal to you for cultivating more reflection in your life?

- What group reflective practices would you like to incorporate in your work setting? What will it take to do this?

- What are your thoughts about the importance of reflection for transforming knowledge into wisdom?

- Identify some ways in which the time Adam the pharmacist spent getting to know Alicia as a person may have saved him (and perhaps other members of the team) time in the long run.

- In what ways did Adam demonstrate wondering about Alicia? In what ways did Adam demonstrate following Alicia? In what ways did he demonstrate holding Alicia?

- In the story, "A Sturdy Presence," is the staff's compassionate care of the man dying of alcoholism something that is likely to happen in the culture in which you work? If so, how are the compassionate values of the people on your team communicated to one another? If you work in a culture where this sort of compassion is not common, what can you as an individual do to influence the culture, or at least to strengthen your own practice?

- Is it easy or difficult for you to stay present with people who are anxious and afraid? What are some things you can do to stay present when others are suffering?

- In "A Sturdy Presence," the family learned later that this nurse's own father had died of alcoholism. What do you think about the nurse's waiting until the patient had passed to let it be known that he'd been through something so similar? When is it helpful to share pieces of your own story with patients and their families and when is it not helpful to do so?

- Recalling the meditation, "So I Get Tired, and I Forget," what kinds of professional experiences tend to make you forget why you went into health care? What kinds of professional experiences help you to remember your purpose and become more energized?

- What do you think of the idea that even when you're tired, you can be there for your patients and their families?

Epilogue:
A Return to Palpation

*When a critical number of people change
how they think and behave, the culture does also . . .
and a new era begins.*

—Jean Shinoda Bolen, psychiatrist

See that lady over there? She's about three minutes away from a diabetic coma. No one else in the room can tell, but I can because I palpate. Because I palpate, I know what to do next.

The little boy in the corner of the playground? He's feeling lost and alone and . . . oh, I didn't see the finger twitching (more data incoming). He might be autistic. He has a specific ailment that means he can't find his way into the group of kids playing. That informs what should be done. I know now that I can't approach him too fast, for example. Were I not a palpator, I wouldn't have known.

Eleanor, the elderly nurse from Ireland, reminded us about palpation in Chapter Four. It's what we do. Some of us have done it since we were children. We know how to get the "feel" of someone or of a social situation or of a problem.

We clinicians are data collectors, nearly always attuned, and we are data synthesizers: we have that incredibly sophisticated, not-everyone-can-do-this capacity for putting the pieces together. We may have learned it as the hyper-responsible child we were in our family of origin. We may have learned it in our professional training; perhaps the science of it appealed to us. The point is we're good at it (or used to be), and it makes for huge efficiencies in our living and in our working.

This book has been about returning to our origins. In medicine, in nursing, and in the allied health professions, we share elements of a common heritage. We attend to others. We are capable of scientific curiosity, including the part about suspending the impulse to reach fixed conclusions and instead continuing the search for understanding. We know how to follow the words of another but also the other's behavior, movements, and affect. We catch on that most people—especially when they're sick, vulnerable, or afraid—need holding, and we have a whole repertoire of holding behaviors.

We've been reminded in this book of a great many things we already knew:

- The provision of health care cannot be done effectively outside of human connection and relatedness.

- Empathy heals wounds.

- Attunement supports the patient's capacity to regulate himself, which improves healing, makes the tasks of data collection and administration of treatment more efficient, and makes our job easier.

- Patients have a great deal to teach us, since there is no one-size-fits-all in health care.

- The ultimate compliment to another human being—indeed, the ultimate intimacy—is to attune to him. Once that happens, we have a bond that significantly increases the likelihood of cooperation.

- Modern, technology-driven health care is marvelous, and at the same time it's a potential impediment to human connection. It's up to us to make technology work for us in the service of human connection.

- The relational aspects of health care are as much a part of our discipline as the instrumental aspects. Healing is threatened if the relational aspect is missing.

What we have tried to stir into the mix of what you already knew are some reminders about how to do it—for those who forgot, who got out of the habit, who never quite understood the components of the relational disciplines, or who are now in a position to teach them to others.

When clinicians are suffering in their work, it's because they're feeling "cut off" from human connection.

As we ask you to remember your purpose in your work, we remember our own purpose in writing this book. In our respective work, both of us talk with countless clinicians in a variety of disciplines. When clinicians are troubled it can be for a variety of reasons, but we see a common denominator in their suffering: They feel disconnected. They're feeling "cut off" from human connection.

The clinician's most compelling reason for focusing on attunement and the therapeutic practices of wondering, following, and holding, is simply that you cannot practice these skills without experiencing human connection. They draw you toward the one thing that can truly nourish you in your work: your moments of presence with other human beings.

It's quite common that clinicians in pain can't easily put their finger on just what it is that's missing, but eventually the same deficit is always discovered. These clinicians may say that they feel alienated from their team, and while they may point to things such as inefficient communication as the problem, their pain comes from a lack of human connection. They may say that they feel as though their patient population has become too challenging, but the pain comes from the feeling that something is impeding their ability to connect human-to-human with their patients. They may feel as though there is too much to do and too little time to do it. Here the pain may come from the fact that they're focusing too much of their attention on the completion of tasks (for which there is literally never enough time), instead of on their connection with people, who often require only a few moments of highly attuned human contact.

Attunement and the therapeutic practices of wondering, following, and holding ensure human connection, and thus the continued nourishment of our patients, their families, and ourselves. However, we do not mean to suggest that this is a two-way relationship in which the clinician gets her emotional needs met. The clinical relationship is a one-way relationship, with the clinician giving to the patient (expecting nothing in return) and the patient receiving from the clinician. That said, when attunement, wondering, following, and holding are practiced, an unavoidable side-effect for the clinician is the experience of human connection.

Attunement and the therapeutic practices of wondering, following, and holding ensure human connection.

Imagine yourself in this scenario (based on Darlington, 2011): You're working as a pediatric specialist caring for the sickest of babies. One of them is now four years old, and has a congenital anomaly that means he has been fed only through a tube since birth. This will likely not change.

The child's dad is overseas in the military. His mother has just given birth to a second child who has the same congenital problem. With two critically ill children, a husband far away, and tremendous financial strain, the mother and children move in with her mother, with whom she has a tense relationship.

One of your colleagues asks you how the mother is coping with all of this. What if this were your answer: "I don't know. I don't have time for that. My job is keeping the baby alive and making sure his mother knows how to do that when I'm not there."

You have just stumbled across a moment of truth that most of us have encountered in our careers in health care. In the morass of overwhelming demands, the press of time, worry about getting basic needs met, and the sometimes life-and-death importance of the instrumental aspects of our job, we sometimes forget to be connected with the human beings in our care. Attunement to a human being gets replaced by a sense of urgency pointed solely toward the technical. We forget to wonder, we aren't quite following, we undervalue holding. We imagine that this is no time for palpation; this is about a baby's immediate needs.

Then, right in the middle of it, we remember the therapeutic practices. We remember that attunement alone has the power to provide some measure of healing for this mother whose daily struggle is beyond our imagining. We remember that the simple practices of wondering, following, and holding—practices that we have now studied and perhaps even applied and reflected upon until we've made them a permanent part of who we are as clinicians—will keep that connection in place during the time we are together and will continue to heal this mother long after our encounter is ended. Is it possible that when this mother has been seen and held for any length of time, she takes a new sense of security with her into everything she does? Could it be that the sense that someone has her back stays with her at least for a while?

So you try again. This time you pause, take the mother aside, and ask: "So, how are *you* doing?" It's not a very complicated question, but you ask it in a way that makes clear that you actually want to know; her answer matters to you. Still, you are surprised when she stares at you for a moment, then bursts into tears. She tells you how overwhelmed, alone, and incompetent she feels. She mentions the dreams of motherhood that have been shattered by the realities of life with these kids. She admits that she has thought about pulling out the baby's feeding tube and letting him die. Your eyes stay connected with hers as you nod slowly, simply receiving her pain and letting it register in you in your own authentic way. You receive her without judgment, and you offer no advice. This is connection for connection's sake, and the healing it provides stands on its own.

Once the human-to-human connection is established (which may or may not have taken an entire minute), everything goes better. You work out some respite and connect the mother with some counseling. The improvement in her efficiency and competence in managing the responsibilities of caring for two critically ill children—along with her mood while doing it—is noticeable right away. She's not afraid of doing something wrong in front of you now that she knows you didn't judge her as she confessed her deepest shame to you. That's when it dawns on you. You've helped someone heal today. You may have saved a baby's life. It took only a few moments. Oddly, your job just got much easier and your visits shorter, because this mother feels much more "on top of it." You know that on this day, you got it right. This is why you entered health care in the first place. Healing happened, and it went beyond what you thought you were there for. People got better, and you had a hand in it.

One of the great blessings of writing this book is that it has forced us to practice what we preach. We've had to test our theories for ourselves, and over the past year we have become almost obsessive observers of attunement, wondering, following, and holding. We have also become keenly aware of the moments in which they are tragically missing. In our observations we have seen with absolute clarity that the clinicians who stay energized in their work are those who feel connected to the human beings around them, while the clinicians who burn out are those who have encountered something in their practice (or in their life outside of their practice) that has interrupted their habit of establishing human connections with the people in their care and the people with whom they work. This loss is as insidious as it is tragic, as it takes hold like a cancer. At first it is small and hidden, but it grows, making its host progressively more tired and weak in the process.

This book is your invitation to do your part to safeguard the heart of first-class practice by deepening your own capacity to engage therapeutically with your patients, their families, and your colleagues. Your individual practice is a contribution to the whole, and it cannot help but change the whole. Just as a butterfly flapping its wings in the Amazon is said to influence the hurricane halfway across the globe, your one moment of human connection has equally profound reverberations.

Your individual practice is a contribution to the whole, and it cannot help but change the whole.

We are concluding this book by calling for a return to palpation—a return to tuning in with intention to the people and situations we encounter. A return to palpation is a return to the senses. It's an invitation to be fully present. We know that this is no small thing to ask even under ideal circumstances. Still, we dare to ask for your presence in the face of human suffering. We invite you to stay connected to the heart of your work and say "yes" to bringing the relational aspects of care to life continually in your daily practice.

Highly attuned therapeutic care is not beyond you. It is in you.

Appendix

Appendix A: Reflecting on Therapeutic Boundaries

Figure A.1 below is adapted from the National Council of State Boards of Nursing, 2004. It is an interesting tool for reflection; as a practice in awareness, we can plot our relationship with any patient and family along the continuum of *over-involvement* to *under-involvement.*

We are over-involved when we seek to have our own needs met through the patient. A simple example of over-involvement is burdening the patient with our feelings of frustration about the workload we're facing or the specific staffing problems on a shift. This takes the focus away from the patient and puts the patient in the position of validating our hardships.

We are under-involved when we see patients as a series of tasks to be completed—as part of our workload for the day—and fail to attune to them as unique people and relate to them therapeutically. We are under-involved when we have little or no interest in who they are, their story, and/or their experience of care. Under-involvement manifests as detached, task-based, routinized care.

FIGURE A.1: Recognizing Therapeutic Boundaries

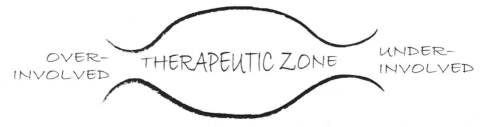

We are in the therapeutic zone when our care is responsive to the patient and family as unique human beings. We wonder about who they are and what this event means to them and to their lives. We follow by listening to their unique story and needs, and we are guided by what they teach us. We hold by being steady and nonjudgmental even in the face of strong emotional responses, and by speaking of patients and their loved ones with respect, always safeguarding their dignity and humanity. Consider these questions in order to gauge your own level of therapeutic involvement:

- In your own practice, in which zone are you most of the time?

- Reflect on a patient/family relationship in which you may have become over-involved. What circumstances make you more likely to move into over-involvement?

- Reflect on a patient/family relationship in which you may have become under-involved. What circumstances make you more likely to move into under-involvement?

- Do you have a colleague who seems particularly adept at maintaining therapeutic boundaries? What does he or she do that you would like to emulate?

Appendix B: Presence and Protocol

In a health care world that is too often driven by procedural protocols, treatment protocols, safety and regulatory protocols, administrative protocols, and even routinization of the morning greeting, what happens to presence?

Such prescribed protocols and other formulaic structures likely originated from a desire for quality care. We wanted to be thorough. We wanted to cover the bases; we wanted to cover our liabilities and to make sure that we were meeting regulatory requirements. We wanted to make sure everyone on the health care team was using the same words to provide consistent messages, which would, we hoped, improve quality, increase safety, and decrease errors.

The necessity of standardization in health care is not in question here. There is no doubt that protocols serve important functions within institutions and organizations. It is the method of their use that we wish to address, particularly in light of what we know about presence and attunement. Simply put, if the protocol is allowed to reduce presence and thus create an obstacle to attunement, our capacity to assess the patient fully is compromised.

Take for example, the admission assessment. Our stated aim is to learn as much about the person as possible, but depending upon who is doing the admission assessment, the process can be far more about completing a form than about learning about a person. People often perceive the clinician's questioning as serving the system, not serving the hallowed purpose of discovering the person and his very personal and very particular health issues. When the patient perceives that the clinician is not fully present and attuned, he may obfuscate, withhold, or give incomplete answers. Suddenly we have jeopardized patient safety (because we are working with incomplete or inaccurate data about the person), exposed the organization to liability (because mistakes are now more likely), and turned the clinician into a stenographer. Patients and families can readily distinguish disinterest and routinization on the part of the clinician, setting the stage for distrust rather than connection.

During one of our daughter's many hospital stays, we listened as resident after resident came in to question her about her condition. Each time, it was the same list of questions from the same written protocol, asked in the same order; the only thing that really changed each time was that it was a different resident making those check marks in those very same boxes. The protocol was allowed to become a barrier to patient-caregiver collaboration. Were those residents there to complete the written protocol or to learn about the person in front of them?

When these sorts of interactions take place, the patient sees the caregiver as serving the organization; she experiences that the caregiver is no longer "with *me*." The breeding ground for patient resentment is created. Satisfaction scores fall. We watched with both embarrassment and empathy as our adolescent daughter began to ignore questions and deny or minimize symptoms because she didn't think the residents were really interested in her. After a while, she didn't see any value in giving them the information, as the residents did not appear to really need or value it.

The protocol itself is not to blame, of course. The culprit is our willingness (episodic or systemic) to allow the protocol to take us away from making a real connection with the people in front of us. In our most hurried moments, we may sacrifice presence in order to complete the protocol.

In the fast-paced, often chaotic world of health care, it's easy to slip into a mindset that encourages us to "just get through it." When we are presented with a routine task such as working through a list of questions or conducting a series of very common tests, we can easily fail to make an authentic connection with the patient. These activities can become so routinized that we may feel we are able to do them in our sleep, and in our most harried moments, we may in fact bring a diminished consciousness to our most routine tasks.

But no task that involves a person can be permitted to become routine—especially a task that could, if done correctly, facilitate gaining greater knowledge and understanding about the patient. Whenever a person is involved, the completion of the most commonplace protocol is elevated to a sacred level.

People cannot be counted on to give us correct, comprehensive, insightful, or even comprehensible answers to our carefully formulated questions. For the patient, health care is a foreign land, so there is almost always a "cultural barrier" that requires us to depart from our formulas in order to follow cues, ask for clarification, and dig deeper to learn what we need to know in order to serve our patients. This deeper digging requires presence. It requires attunement with the patient. It requires that we wonder about our patients and that we invite them into wondering with us on their behalf. It requires that we follow the cues they give us, and ask more when we sense something beneath the surface that we want to see more clearly. It requires that we hold the patient with dignity, even in the accomplishment of tasks that are, for us, completely commonplace.

The point of working from a prescribed list of questions is, of course, to be complete and accurate in gathering information. However, when our goal becomes just completing the document, we are no longer invested in learning about the patient as a whole person. Here, a conundrum in health care emerges. When audits are conducted, the clinician will not be asked what he or she knows about any particular patient; instead, compliance is determined by whether or not every box on the form is completed. Time allotted for learning about patients is already limited, and it seems to be constantly shrinking. We work within a system that does not make it easy for the clinician to make room for attunement or presence. The perception of dwindling time presents a challenge to health care clinicians.

More often than not, however, we meet the challenge brilliantly. Here are some of the ways we remain present despite time constraints and repetitive protocols:

- We maintain eye contact, never allowing the computer or the printed protocol to come between us and the person in front of us—the one we are present with.

- We share the computer screen with the patient, allowing her to view the questions, protocols, and responses.

- We use contingent communication, following up on answers—or even inflections—with new questions or new versions of the question already asked.

- We convey in words and body language that we are more interested in the person than the task—that the purpose of the task is to serve the person in our care.

- We explain to the patient the process of capturing her story, keeping it safe and available for the next clinician.

More often than not, we do not choose between protocols and presence; instead we combine the two, intentionally crafting a way to optimize the potential of each to excellent effect. Systems and protocols used within our organizations are tools that facilitate our care. These tools, when used with flexibility and the goal of acquiring information and discovering another human being, help us to work more effectively. When we are the masters of our tools, the efficacy of our work increases dramatically, but when we become slaves to our tools, we may disengage emotionally from our patients (Barager, 2011), and no one benefits—not the patient, not the clinician, and not the organization that put the tools into our hands.

Caregivers know how to create connection with the patient as the first order of business. Caregivers connect by being present, by remaining curious about the person rather than drawing swift conclusions, by following the person's verbal and non-verbal cues, and by asking the questions on the admission form in a way that safeguards the person's dignity, and then asking additional questions—questions so patient-specific that no protocol could possibly predict them—in a way that supports and enhances the connection and promotes care and safety.

Appendix C: Kleinmann's Eight Questions

The Eight Questions:

1. What do you call the problem (the illness, the reason you or your family member is in the hospital, etc.)?

2. What do you think has caused the problem (what has made this illness appear)?

3. Why do you think it started when it did? (an important difference from "How long has this been going on?")

4. What do you think the sickness does? How does it work?

5. How severe is the sickness? Will it have a short or a long course?

6. What kind of treatment do you think that you or your family member should receive? What are the most important results you hope for from this treatment?

7. What are the chief problems the sickness has caused?

8. What do you fear most about the sickness?

Adapted from Kleinman, A. et al (1978). Culture, illness and care: Clinical lessons from anthropologic and cross-cultural research. *Annals of Internal Medicine, 88,* 251-288.

Appendix D: "I Didn't Do Anything Wrong, so Why do I Have to Apologize?"

Apologizing seems to have become increasingly misunderstood. Lawyers advise against saying, "I'm sorry," even when saying it might end the threat of a lawsuit. "If you say you're sorry, you're admitting culpability," a cautious attorney might reasonably suggest. "Do you want to hear that played back in court?"

A simple human overture has been turned into a weapon, and the withholding of it, turned into a defense. Over time, our collective fear of expressing sincere regret due to fear of liability has resulted in health care cultures in which defensiveness prevails. There was a time when it was standard practice not to inform patients about medical errors (Singer, 2010). However, leading health care organizations are now recognizing that apologies work for everyone involved—not just for the injured person, but for health care professionals themselves. Doug Wojcieszak founded an organization called Sorry Works which is dedicated to helping health care professionals, legal professionals, and insurance companies work through crises resulting from medical errors and negligence. Wojcieszak, whose brother died in 1998 because of medical errors, experienced what he calls the "typical cover-up": a wall of silence, avoidance, and defensiveness. His organization's mission is to help professionals understand the importance of empathy and apology in painful situations (Syme, 2012).

But it's not just in health care that "I'm sorry" can be so terribly complicated. Some couples abuse the words, apologizing when they don't mean it just to end the conversation. One may say, "I'm sorry" sideways, as in: "I'm sorry you heard that," or "I'm sorry if you let yourself be hurt by that." It sounds sincere initially, but ten minutes later it hits you that "I'm very sorry your feelings are hurt" sounds more like an accusation that you're oversensitive than an actual apology.

What oppresses us is the inappropriate linkage we make between a genuine, empathetic remark of regret—of expressing that one is disturbed by the pain of another—and declaring that one is at fault for that pain. An apology is not an admission of culpability; it's an expression of empathetic validation for one who is hurting.

Perhaps it will help to consider the idea of who an apology is really for. The term "service recovery" is used to describe an apology meant to put a person or institution back into the good graces of someone who has been let down in some way while in our care. Service recovery apologies have a specific purpose, and it isn't to help the other person actually feel better. The aim of a service recovery apology is to alter the perception of the person so that the clinician or institution is seen in a more flattering light by those who will ultimately be filling out an evaluation of the care. This kind of apology is likely to be ineffective because nearly anyone on the receiving end can see that it is offered in a self-serving, self-protecting way. The one offering the apology isn't conveying that he is "disturbed by the pain of the other"; he is conveying that he is disturbed by the idea that the other might think ill of him or his organization.

An authentic apology is not about altering the perception of another person. The goal of an authentic apology is to ease the other's pain by acknowledging it, thus facilitating the other's healing. In a therapeutic interaction, the aim is to restore the patient's sense of balance, optimism, and trust—not so that we will be *seen* as an institution that promotes balance, optimism and trust, but so that the patient might heal.

As British writer G.K. Chesterton famously wrote, "The injured party does not want to be compensated because he has been wronged; he wants to be healed because he has been hurt."

It should not matter that it could be solely the patient's perception that he's been let down in our care. Most often something has occurred to create that perception, and often that something is influenced by, or within the control of, the clinician. Patient discontent is often related to an unmet need, to physical and/or emotional pain, to missed communication, and/or to a failure to deliver what we've promised. Health care providers are charged with the complex work of understanding the source of the patient's discontent, naming that discontent, talking about it, and then taking action to help the patient recover from it.

Sincere apology acknowledges the pain of the other and seeks to understand what might be done to ease that pain. In our experience, there are four things we can do to facilitate healing in one who is feeling dropped in our care:

- We can offer our presence, providing the person our undivided attention.

- We can attune to the person, breathing deeply, regulating our body, mind, and spirit to meet the other where she is, and then be a steady, caring, healing presence for her.

- We can wonder with our patients and on their behalf, being curious with them as their stories unfold.

- We can follow what our patients convey to us, both verbally and nonverbally, by using all the information they give us to help facilitate their mental, emotional, and spiritual recovery.

The words of a truly healing apology needn't be complicated. When clinicians are present and attuned as they wonder on behalf of the patient and follow his cues closely, his discomfort can be alleviated in a moment. When a clinician says something as simple as, "I am so sorry," perhaps followed by,

"Help me understand what's going on here," the apology serves the other. If the clinician seeks to acknowledge the suffering of the other, to listen closely, and to understand, the apology creates a moment of healing for the patient.

We needn't be obsequious about apologizing, nor do we need to do it too often. Indeed, the earnestness of our acknowledgment of the other's injury is all the richer for the rarity of its expression. But what a marvelous experience it can be for the one who hurts, to hear another join in the hurt long enough to say, "I'm sorry."

The size of the hurt does not matter. The irritable patient who complains that the coffee on her dinner tray is cold may appear to be upset over a minor slight, but a slight it is, nonetheless—and to this patient, at this moment, with nothing going right, feeling acutely how few things can be made right, it seems like a significant offense. It hurts, and our job is to tend to what hurts. It's amazing what an earnest acknowledgment can mean at that moment: "I'll bet cold coffee is the last thing you wanted. I am so sorry."

All things considered, an apology is an incredibly efficient intervention—with our children, with our neighbors, with a stranger whose car we bumped, and with a best friend whose mother is ill. An authentic apology is, in essence, a therapeutic action that can alleviate pain and facilitate healing.

In order to be able to apologize authentically, you must have a sense of how apology works (or does not work) in your current practice. We invite you to reflect on these questions:

- Is it easy or difficult for me to apologize?

- If apology is easy for me, who are my apologies for? What are they typically designed to do?

- If apology is hard for me, what is my definition of apology? What are my feelings about people who easily say they're sorry?

- What would it take for me to rethink my current relationship with apology to make it more deliberate and completely authentic?

Authentic apologies demonstrate that we really do care and that we are interested in restoring relationships. The act of restoring relationships provides the possibility of winning back the trust of the person whose faith in us was shaken. The trust of our patients matters, not because we want to be in the good graces of our patients, but because the person who trusts us is going to have a far more comfortable time of it than the person who is nervously watchful, expecting us to fail.

It's common among clinicians, when encouraged to apologize, to protest, "I didn't do anything wrong, so why do I have to apologize?" Our answer is, "Why would you hesitate to apologize if you did nothing wrong?" Your apology may help to ease the discomfort of the other. If you're blameless in the midst of a snafu, an apology can help, but it can't hurt. When we understand our own relationship with apology, as well as what it can mean to our relationships with patients, their families, and our colleagues, apologizing may become a practical and potent part of our therapeutic practice.

Appendix E: How Health Care Organizations can be Aligned to Consistently Put Patients and their Families First

There are many examples of extraordinary organizational commitment to transforming health care cultures to provide humane and compassionate patient care. These organizations seek to design and implement the best possible systems and provide the best possible leadership to support clinical staff, physicians, and patients and families.

While organizational transformation is outside of the scope of this book, we would be remiss if we didn't highlight some of the factors that facilitate successful organizational change. Such change must be made in order to support the clinician-patient relationship. We have found that successful organizational transformations include the following success factors (Chapman, 2003; Frampton, Gilpin, & Charmel, 2003; Gerteis, Edgman-Levitan, Daley & Delbanco, 2002; Kolo-troutis, 2004; Studer, 2006):

- **Executive commitment:** At the executive and board level, there is a clear and compelling commitment to the mission of serving patients and families in a holistic way. These organizations have explicitly named their commitment to keeping patients and families in the center of all of their planning and design.

- **Leadership throughout the organization:** There is a mindset among the executive team and all positional leaders that leadership is a quality that can be found within everyone in the organization. The leaders think inclusively rather than hierarchically and understand that commitment is more valuable than compliance. Decision making is placed in the hands of those affected by the decisions.

- **Sustained focus:** During tough times, these organizations remain focused on the mission and do not throw away those things that are critical to supporting excellence in patient care and service. They use change management methodologies that ensure that they don't lose focus on their mission even through a long transition with many twists and turns along the way.

- **Valuing improvement of the patient's experience above all else:** Qualitative outcomes are valued along with quantitative measures. Visible improvement of the patient and family experience is inspiring to physicians and staff at all levels and will result in improvement in patient satisfaction scores. However, the scores are the byproduct rather than the focus of the efforts. The leaders understand that in order to have high patient satisfaction scores, the organization must develop and nurture compassionate relationships throughout the organization as well as with patients and families.

- **Reflection and educational development:** Organizations that experience successful transformations invest in the development of their people. Leaders believe that learning is critical to excellence in patient care. These organizations devote time to reflection and dialogue about best practices in patient care, team work, and what it takes to inspire and sustain high-performing cultures.

- **Visible, accessible leaders:** Positional leaders are visible within the organization and they are accessible to everyone. Information is shared, doors are open, and leaders seek wisdom from people throughout the organization, regardless of position. There is an attitude of "we're in this together."

- **Trust and integrity are consistently demonstrated:** Leaders and committees do what they say they'll do in the short run and over the long haul, and their results are made visible throughout the organization. Their behaviors align with their stated values and beliefs.

- **Building relationships:** A culture is created in which relationships are built and nurtured every step of the way. If relationship building between clinicians and patients is a core value, relationship building must also be a visible value that is demonstrated everywhere in the organization—among the nursing staff, between physicians and nurses, etc.—so that everyone is moving as a whole organization toward a common goal.

Appendix F: Recognizing Compassion Fatigue

Symptoms of compassion fatigue can be highly disruptive, and yet if they are recognized and become a catalyst for positive change, the results can be transformative. While there is no easy fix, if individuals and teams make a decision to recognize the symptoms and to take strong and positive action for change, a new level of awareness, resiliency and capacity to thrive is achievable (Compassion Fatigue Awareness Project, 2012).

The Thriving Scale is a simple tool we use to bring to the surface awareness of the current state of well-being of an individual, team, or organizational culture. Health care clinicians are accustomed to the self-reported pain intensity scale. The Thriving Scale is a simple reverse of that, with *Thriving*, the highest state of well-being, scored at a 10 and *Compassion Fatigue*, the lowest state of well-being, scored at a 1. *Surviving* is in the middle of the scale. This continuum can be used to assess oneself or to invite dialogue among members of a group. If we don't wonder about our own state of well-being or that of our colleagues, and if we don't inquire about it, we have no way of taking informed, positive action for greater health and well-being throughout our organization. If we don't tend to our own health, we cannot be effective in caring for the health of our patients.

Thriving Scale

Compassion Fatigue			Surviving				Thriving		
1	2	3	4	5	6	7	8	9	10
A chronic clouding of caring and concern for others; physical, emotional, and spiritual exhaustion; decreased ability to experience joy			Endure, live through, persist, pull through, breathe, continue, do, go on, prevail, stay, cope				Do well, flourish, grow, shine, radiate, develop, get ahead, be abundant, connect with others		

- Where on the scale do you see yourself currently (at least 80% of the time)?

- Where on the scale would you rate your team as a whole (at least 80% of the time)?

- Where would you rate your work culture currently (at least 80% of the time)?

- What is one thing that you could integrate into your practice immediately that would move you closer to thriving?

The Compassion Fatigue Awareness Project (2012) is an important resource for understanding and resolving compassion fatigue. They identify the symptoms of compassion fatigue both for the individual and for the organization.

Compassion Fatigue Symptoms Present in an Individual

- Excessive blaming

- Bottled-up emotions

- Isolation from others

- Receives an unusual number of complaints from others

- Voices excessive complaints about administrative functions

- Substance abuse

- Compulsive behaviors such as overspending, overeating, gambling, sexual addiction

- Poor self-care (e.g., hygiene, appearance)

- Legal problems, indebtedness

- Recurring nightmares about and/or flashbacks to traumatic events

- Chronic physical ailments such as gastrointestinal problems and recurring colds

- Apathetic, sad, no longer finds activities pleasurable

- Difficulty concentrating

- Mentally and physically tired

- Preoccupied

- In denial about problems

When compassion fatigue becomes prevalent within the workplace, the organization as a whole suffers ill health, often characterized by chronic absenteeism, rising worker's compensation costs, high turnover rates, conflict between employees, low engagement scores, physician dissatisfaction, patient and family dissatisfaction, and a culture of mistrust and lack of respect.

Symptoms of Organizational Compassion Fatigue:

- High absenteeism

- Constant changes in co-worker relationships

- Inability of teams to work well together

- Desire among staff members to break company rules

- Aggressive behaviors among staff

- Inability of staff to complete assignments and tasks

- Inability of staff to meet deadlines

- Lack of flexibility among staff members

- Negativity towards management

- Strong reluctance to change

- Inability of staff to believe that improvement is possible

- Lack of a vision for the future.

Organizations tend to know when they're suffering from organizational compassion fatigue. Even before their patient satisfaction scores drop, they have a sense that the wheels have come off—complaints increase, problems mount, and answers don't come easily.

Adapted with permission from "Recognizing Compassion Fatigue" by Compassion Fatigue Awareness Project © 2012.

References

Ackoff, R. L. (1989). From data to wisdom. *Journal of Applied Systems Analysis, 16*(1), 3-9.

Arbinger Institute. (2006). *The anatomy of peace: Resolving the heart of conflict.* San Francisco: Berrett-Koehler.

Argyris, C. (2008). *Teaching smart people how to learn.* Boston: Harvard Business Press.

Austin, W. (2011). The incommensurability of nursing as a practice and the customer service model: An evolutionary threat to the discipline. Nursing Philosophy, 12, 158-166.

Baldwin, C., & Linnea, A. (2010). *The circle way: A leader in every chair.* San Francisco: Berrett-Koehler Publishers, Inc.

Baldwin, C. (1998). *Calling the circle.* New York: Bantam Books.

Barager, R., KevinMD. (2011, April). Re: How an EMR emotionally disengages physicians from their patients [Web log post]. Retrieved from http://www.kevinmd.com/blog/2011/04/emr-emotionally-disengages-physicians-patients.html

Becker-Weidman, A., & Shell, D. (2010). *Attachment parenting: Developing connections and healing children.* Lanham, MD: Jason Aronson.

Benner, P., Sutphen, M., Leonard, V., & Day, L. (2010). *Educating nurses: A call for radical transformation.* Stanford, CA: Carnegie Foundation for the Advancement of Teaching.

Blakeslee, S. (2006, January 10). Cells that read minds. *The New York Times*, pp. F1, F4.

Block, P. (2002). *The answer to how is yes: Acting on what matters.* San Francisco: Berrett-Koehler.

Blum, D. (2002). *Love at Goon Park: Harry Harlow and the science of affection.* Cambridge, MA: Perseus Books.

Bolte Taylor, J. (2006). *My stroke of insight: A brain scientist's personal journey.* New York: Penguin Press.

Bowen, M., & Kerr, M. (1988). *Family evaluation.* New York: Norton and Company.

Bowlby, J. (1958). The nature of the child's tie to his mother. *International Journal of Psychoanalysis, 39,* 350-373.

Bowlby, J. (1969). *Attachment and loss series, volume I: Attachment.* New York: Basic Books.

Brafman, O., & Brafman, R. (2010). *Click: The magic of instant connections.* New York: Broadway Books.

Brazelton, T.B., & Cramer, B. (1990). *The earliest relationship: Parents, infants, and the drama of early attachment.* New York: Addison-Wesley Publishing Co.

Brooks, J. L. (Producer), & Brooks, J. L. (Director). (1983). *Terms of endearment* [Motion picture]. United States: Paramount Pictures.

Brown, B. (2010). *The power of vulnerability* [Video file]. Retrieved from http://www.ted.com/talks/brene_brown_on_vulnerability.html

Brown, B. (2012, March). *Listening to shame* [Video file]. Retrieved from http://www.ted.com/talks/brene_brown_listening_to_shame.html

Buber, M. (1958). *I and thou.* New York: Scribner's.

Bush, E. (2001). The use of human touch to improve the well-being of older adults: A holistic nursing intervention. *Journal of Holistic Nursing, 19,* 256-270.

Bush, H. (2011, December). Doubling down on the patient experience. *Hospitals and Health Networks,* 23-25.

Chamberlain, D. (1998). *The mind of your newborn baby.* Berkeley: North Atlantic Books.

Chapman, E. (2007). *Radical loving care: Building the healing hospital in America.* Nashville, TN: Erie Chapman Foundation.

REFERENCES

Charon, R. (2004). The ethicality of narrative medicine. In Hurwitz, B., Greenhalgh, T., & Skultans, V. (Eds.), *Narrative Research in Health and Illness* (pp. 23-25). Retrieved from http://onlinelibrary.wiley.com/book/10.1002/9780470755167

Charon, R. (2006). *Narrative medicine: Honoring the stories of illness.* New York: Oxford University Press.

Compassion Fatigue Awareness Project. (2012). *Recognizing compassion fatigue.* Retrieved from www.compassionfatigue.org

Cooperrider, D., & Whitney, D. (2007). Appreciative Inquiry: A positive revolution in change. In Holman, P., & Devane, T. (Eds.), *The change handbook* (pp. 245-263). San Francisco: Berrett-Koehler.

Covey, S. (1989). *The seven habits of highly successful people: Powerful lessons in personal change.* New York: Simon and Schuster.

Damasio, A. (1994). *Descartes' error: Emotion, reason and the human brain.* New York: Quill.

Damasio, A. (2003). *Looking for Spinoza: Joy, sorrow and the feeling brain.* Orlando, FL: Harcourt.

Darlington, N. (2011, Fall). Keeping a lookout: Being aware of opportunities to support parent/child relationships. *Everyday's Child, 21,* 1-2.

Dickey, L., Truten, J., Gross, L., Deitrick, L. (2011). Promotion of staff resiliency and interdisciplinary team cohesion through two small-group narrative exchange models designed to facilitate patient-and family-centered care. *Journal of Communication in Healthcare, 4*(2), 126-138.

Eberman, L. (2010). Enhancing clinical evaluation skills: Palpation as the principal skill. *Athletic Training Education Journal, 5*(4), 170-175.

Emde, R., & Sorce, J. (1983). The rewards of infancy: Emotional availability and maternal referencing. In Call, J., Galenson, E., & Tyson, R. (Eds.), *Frontiers of Infant Psychiatry* (pp. 17-30). New York: Basic Books,

Engel, M. (2010). *I'm here: Compassionate communication in patient care.* Orlando, FL: Phillips Press.

Felgen, J. (2004). A caring and healing environment. In M. Koloroutis (Ed.), *Relationship-based care: A model for transforming practice* (pp. 23-52). Minneapolis, MN: Creative Health Care Management.

411

Ferguson, S. (Producer), & Jackson, M. (Director). (2010). *Temple Grandin* [TV]. United States: HBO.

Field, T. (Ed.). (1995). *Touch in early development.* Mahwah, NJ: Lawrence Erlbaum Associates, Inc.

Figley, C. R. (Ed.). (1995). *Compassion fatigue: Coping with secondary traumatic stress disorder in those who treat the traumatized.* New York: Brunner/Mazel.

Frampton, S., Gilpin, L., & Charmel, P. (2003). *Putting patients first: Designing and practicing patient-centered care.* San Francisco: Jossey-Bass.

Gerteis, M., Edgman-Levitan, S., Daley, J., & Delbanco, T. (Eds.). (2002). *Through the*

patient's eyes: Understanding and promoting patient-centered care. San Francisco: Jossey-Bass.

Gianino, A., & Tronick, E. Z. (1988). The mutual regulation model: The infant's self and interactive regulation, coping and defense. In Field, T., McCabe, P., & Schneiderman, N. (Eds.), *Stress and coping.* Hillsdale, NJ: Erlbaum.

Gorlick, A. (2009, August 24). Media multitaskers pay mental price, Stanford study shows. Retrieved from http://news.stanford.edu/news/2009/august24/ multitask-research-study-082409.html

Groves, J. (1978). Taking care of the hateful patient. *New England Journal of Medicine, 298*, 883-887.

Hughes, D. (2007). *Building the bonds of attachment: Awakening love in deeply troubled children* (2nd ed.). Lanham, MD: Jason Aronson.

Hughes, D. (2009). *Attachment-focused parenting: Effective strategies to care for children.* New York: W.W. Norton.

Joinson, C. (1992). Coping with compassion fatigue. *Nursing 22*(4), 116-122.

Jourard, S. (1971). *The transparent self.* (2nd ed.). New York: Von Nostrand Reinhold Co.

Jung, C. (1957). *The undiscovered self.* Florence, KY: Routledge.

Keck, G., & Kupecky, R. (1995). *Adopting the hurt child: Hope for families with special-needs kids.* Colorado Springs: Pinon Press.

Kleinman, A., Eisenberg L., & Good, B. (1978). Culture, illness and care: Clinical lessons from anthropologic and cross-cultural research. *Annals of Internal Medicine, 88,* 251-258.

Koloroutis, M. (2009). *Re-igniting the spirit of caring participant manual* (2nd ed.). Minneapolis, MN: Creative Health Care Management.

Koloroutis, M. (Ed.). (2004). *Relationship-based care: A model for transforming practice.* Minneapolis, MN: Creative Health Care Management.

Koloroutis, M., Felgen, J., Person, C., & Wessel, S. (Eds.). (2007). *Relationship-Based Care field guide.* Minneapolis, MN: Creative Health Care Management.

Kovacs, P., Bellin, M. H., & Fauri, D. (2006). Family-centered care. *Journal of Social Work in End-Of-Life & Palliative Care, 2*(1), 13–27.

Kunc, N., & Van der Klift, E. (Producers). (1995). *A credo for support* [DVD]. United States: Broadreach Training & Resources.

Langer, E. (1997). *The power of mindful learning.* Cambridge, MA: Da Capo Press.

LarryBrownSports. (2010, April 6). Re: Da'Sean Butler apologized to Bob Huggins for letting him down [Web log post]. Retrieved from http://larrybrownsports.com/college-basketball/dasean-butler-halftime-interview-bob-huggins/15387

Lawler, J. (1993). *Behind the screens: Nursing, somology, and the problem of the body.* Redwood City, CA: The Benjamin/Cummings Publishing Company.

LeMaistre, J. (1985). *Beyond rage: The emotional impact of chronic physical illness.* Oak Park, Illinois: Alpine Guild, Inc.

Levine, S. (1998). *A year to live: How to live this year as if it were your last.* New York: Bell Tower.

Levy, T., & Orlans, M. (1998). *Attachment, trauma and healing: Understanding and treating attachment disorder in children and families.* Washington, DC: Child Welfare League of America Press.

Lown, B. (January, 2007). Difficult conversations: Anger in the clinician-patient/family relationship. *Southern Medical Journal, 100*(1), pp. 34-39.

Falcone, L. M., & Lynn, J. (Producers), & Garcia, R. (Director). (2009). *Mother and child* [Motion picture]. United States: Sony Pictures Classics.

Main, M., Kaplan, N., & Cassidy, J. (1985). Security in infancy, childhood, and adulthood: A move to the level of representation. In Bretherton, I., & Waters, E. (Eds.), *Monographs of the Society for Research in Child Development*, *50*(1), pp. 66-104. Ann Arbor, MI: The Society for Research in Child Development, Inc.

Mann, E. (Producer), & Fishman, B. (Director). (2010, April 3). *NCAA playoffs: West Virginia v. Duke* [TV]. United States: CBS Sports.

Manthey, M. (2007). *What is a nursing salon?* Retrieved from http://mariesnursingsalon.wordpress.com/

Manthey, M. (2010). A new model of healing for the profession of nursing. *Creative Nursing Journal*, *16*(1), 19.

Nathanielsz, P. (2001). *The prenatal prescription.* New York: HarperCollins.

Neubauer, P., & Neubauer, A. (1990). *Nature's thumbprint: The new genetics of personality.* Reading, MA: Addison-Wesley Publishing.

Nhat Hanh, T. (1992). *Peace is every step: The path of mindfulness in everyday life.* New York: Bantam Books.

Nichols, M.P. (1995). *The lost art of listening.* New York: Guilford Press.

Ophir, E., Nass, C., & Wagner, A. D. (2009). Cognitive control in media multitaskers. *Proceedings of the National Academy of Sciences of the United States of America. 106*, 15583-15587. doi:10.1073_pnas.0903620106

Ornish, D. (1997). *Love and survival: The scientific basis for the healing power of intimacy.* New York: HarperCollins.

Parelli, P. (2012). Seven keys to success with the Parelli method of natural horse training. Retrieved from http://www.parellinaturalhorsetraining.com/seven-keys-success/

Peck, M. S. (1987). *The different drum: Community making and peace.* New York: Simon & Schuster.

Pfifferling, J., & Gilley, K. (2000). Overcoming compassion fatigue. *Family Practice Management*, *7*(4), 39-44.

Piercy, M. (2010). *The hunger moon: New and selected poems, 1980-2010.* New York: Alfred A. Knopf.

REFERENCES

Plaas, K. (2002). Like a bunch of cattle: The patient's experience of the outpatient health care environment. In S.P. Thomas & H.R. Pollio (Eds.), *Listening to patients: A phenomenological approach to nursing research and practice* (pp. 237-251). New York: Springer Publishing.

Pruett, K. (1984). A chronology of defensive adaptations to severe psychological trauma. *Psychoanalytic Study of the Child, 39,* 591-612.

Rechtschaffen, S. (1996). *Time shifting: Creating more time to enjoy your life.* New York: Doubleday.

Remen, R. N. (2002, September/October). Re: Interview by Dennis Hughes. *Share Guide.* Retrieved from http://www.shareguide.com/Remen.html

Remen, R. N. (1989). The search for healing. In R. Carlson & B. Shield (Eds.), *Healers on healing* (pp. 91-96). New York: Penguin Putnam, Inc.

Remen, R. N. (1996). *Kitchen table wisdom: Stories that heal.* New York: The Berkley Publishing Group.

Rizzolatti, G., Fogassi, L., & Gallese, V. (2001). Neurophysiological mechanisms underlying the understanding and imitation of action. *Nature Reviews Neuroscience, 2,* 661-670.

Rogers, Carl. (1951). *Client-centered therapy: Its current practice, implications and theory.* London: Constable.

Rotter, J.B. (1954). *Social learning and clinical psychology.* New York: Prentice-Hall.

Sanghavi, D. (2006). What makes for a compassionate patient-caregiver relationship? *Journal on Quality and Patient Safety, 32*(5), 283-292.

Savett, L. (2002). *The human side of medicine: Learning what it's like to be a patient and what it's like to be a physician.* Westport, CT: Auburn House.

Schön, D. (1987). *Educating the reflective practitioner.* San Francisco: John Wiley and Sons, Inc.

Schore, A. (2001). Minds in the making: Attachment, the self-organizing brain, and developmentally-oriented psychoanalytic psychotherapy. *British Journal of Psychotherapy, 17*(3), 299-328.

Schore, A. (2002). The neurobiology of attachment and early personality organization. *Journal of Prenatal and Perinatal Psychology and Health, 16*(3), 249-263.

Schuster N. D., Nelson D.L., & Quisling C. (1984, March). Burnout among physical therapists. *Journal of the American Physical Therapy Association, 64*(3) 299-303.

Shattell, M., & Hogan, B. (2005). Facilitating communication: How to truly understand what patients mean. *Journal of Psychosocial Nursing and Mental Health Services, 43*(10), 29-32.

Siegel, D. (1999). *The developing mind: Toward a neurobiology of interpersonal experience.* New York: The Guilford Press.

Siegel, D. (2007). *The mindful brain: Reflection and attunement in the cultivation of well-being.* New York: W.W. Norton.

Sinclair, L. (2007, Spring). Interview with Rita Charon. *Synapse 3*(1). Retrieved from http://www.mainehumanities.org/programs/litandmed/synapse/insideout_s07.html

Singer, N. (January 9, 2012) Is 'sorry' the hardest word in health care? *The New York Times.* Retrieved from http://www.nytimes.com/2010/01/10/business/10stream.html?_r=1

Smith, M.E., & Hart, G. (1994, October). Nurses' responses to patient anger: From disconnecting to connecting. *Journal of Advanced Nursing, 20*(4) 643-51.

Strain, J. (1979). Psychological reactions to chronic medical illness. *Psychiatric Quarterly, 51*(3), 179-183.

Studer, Q. (2006). *Hardwiring excellence: Purpose, worthwhile work, making a difference.* Gulf Breeze, FL: Fire Starter Publishing.

Swanson, K. (1991). Empirical development of a middle range theory of caring. *Nursing Research, 40*(3), 161-166.

Swanson, K. (1993). Nursing as informed caring for the well-being of others. *IMAGE: Journal of Nursing Scholarship, 25*(4) 352-357.

Swanson, K. (2007). Enhancing nurses' capacity for compassionate caring. In M. Koloroutis, J. Felgen, C. Person, & S. Wessel (Eds.), *Relationship-Based Care field guide* (pp. 502-507). Minneapolis, MN: Creative Health Care Management.

Syme, C. (June 7, 2012) *Sorry works! Helping healthcare deal with crisis.* Retrieved from http://cksyme.org/sorry-works-helping-healthcare-deal-with-crisis

The Schwartz Center For Compassionate Healthcare. (2011, Fall/Winter). New Schwartz Center Rounds sites. *Touchpoints,* 5. Retrieved from http://www.theschwartzcenter.org/pageFiles/1U73WJ4AET1K7YF.pdf

REFERENCES

The Schwartz Center For Compassionate Healthcare. (2012). *Research supports the importance of compassionate, patient-centered care.* Retrieved from http://www. theschwartzcenter.org/pageFiles/B8QX76CRNAWSJU7.pdf

Thomas S. P., & Pollio, H. (2002). *Listening to patients: A phenomenological approach to nursing research and practice.* New York: Springer.

Thomas, S. (2003). Anger: The mismanaged emotion. *Medsurg Nursing, 12*(2), 103-110.

Tronick, E., & Cohn, J. F. (1989). Infant-mother face-to-face interaction: Age and gender difference in coordination and the occurrence of miscoordination. *Child Development, 60*(1), 85-92.

Trout, M. (1993). *Operating principle of the Infant-Parent Institute.* Champaign, IL: The Infant-Parent Institute.

Trout, M. (2011). *See me as a person: Meditations for deepening and sustaining Relationship-Based Care* [CD]. Minneapolis, MN: Creative Health Care Management.

Trout, M., & Thomas, L. (2005). *The Jonathon letters: One family's use of support as they took in, and fell in love with, a troubled child.* Champaign, IL: The Infant-Parent Institute.

Trout, M. (2011). Presence and attunement in health care: A view from infancy research. *Creative Nursing, 17*(1), 16-21.

The University of Kansas Hospital. (2010, April 7). Sitting down on the job: New data finds that patients are happier when doctors sit down, even if they don't stay as long. [News release]. Retrieved from http://www.kumed.com/ newsroom/news/patients-happier-when-doctors-sit-down

Vogt, E., Brown, J., & Isaacs, D. (2003). *The art of powerful questions: Catalyzing insight, innovation, and action.* Mill Valley, CA: Whole Systems Associates.

Warner, C.T. (2001). *Bonds that make us free: Healing our relationships, coming to ourselves.* Nashville, TN: Shadow Mountain Publishing.

Watson, J. (1988). *Nursing: Human science and human care, a theory of nursing.* Sudbury, MA: National League for Nursing.

Watson, J. (1999). *Postmodern nursing and beyond.* Edinburgh, Scotland: Churchill Livingstone/WB Saunders.

Watson, J. (2005). The Caring Moment. On *Care for the journey* [CD]. Novato, CA: Companion Arts/Wisdom of the World.

Watson, J. (2008). *Nursing: The philosophy and science of caring.* (Rev. ed.). Boulder: University Press of Colorado.

Weil, S. (2009). *Waiting for God* (E. Craufurd, Trans.). New York: Harper Perennial Modern Classics (Reprinted from 1951, New York: G. P. Putnam's Sons). Retrieved from http://books.google.com

Wheatley, M. (2010).When did we forget this? In Baldwin, C., & Linnea, A., *The circle way: A leader in every chair.* (p. ix).San Francisco: Berrett-Koehler.

Williamson, M. (1994). *Illuminata: A return to prayer.* New York: Berkley Publishing Group.

Index

H

hand washing, 87, 268, 316, 326–27, 343, 345

Hart, G., 294

HCAHPS (Hospital Consumer Assessment of Healthcare Providers and Systems), 7

healing vs. curing, 17, 29–30, 69

healing/healing presence
  applying palpation to, 379–86
  contrast of "split" and "robotic," 81–82
  obstacles to conscious listening, 149–53
  providing compassionate witness, 188–90
  role of apology in, 396–400
  summary of key points, 88, 90

health care industry
  accountability and measurable outcomes, xi, 15
  chaotic care environments, 246–49
  description of "ideal patient," 218
  including palpation in, 379–86
  nursing as a culture, not just a job, 362
  obstacles to patient care, 241–45
  organizational culture, 245–46, 401
  patients as customers, xi–xii, 6–11, 34–35
  protocols and standardization, 390–94
  putting patients and family first, 401–03

health care provider/team
  about purposes of this book, 16
  anger, dealing with, 294–99
  aspects of clinical practice, 311–13
  carrying the mantle of expertise, 115
  clinician defined, 16
  expectations and standards, 261, 390
  families as members of, xiii, 209–13, 217–27
  feelings of devotion to patients, 177–79
  functioning in a chaotic environment, 255–57
  holding, importance of, 183–85
  holding in crisis situations, 197–200
  learning to support each other, 245–46

patient connectedness and, 204–06
patient disconnectedness and, 206–09, 213–17
reflection and dialogue, 235–37, 245–46, 402
self-assessment, 258–59
team assessment, 263–66
time constraints, 266–79

heart disease, 110–12

"Her Name Was Ruth" (Trout), 185–88

Hockett, Dylan, 297

hold/holding (creating a safe haven)
  about the meaning and purpose of, x–xi
  about the process/meaning of, 3–5
  applying palpation to, 379–86
  author meditation on power of, 185–88
  basic overview of chapter, 18–19
  creating a therapeutic mindset, 48–49
  creating connection, 203–06
  creating disconnection, 206–09
  defined/described, 179–82
  discernment vs. scripted behavior, 182–83
  expectations and requirements, 183–85
  family role in, 217–27
  feelings of devotion to patients, 177–79
  in times of anger, 201–03
  in times of crisis, 197–201
  phases of the process, 190–97
  providing compassionate witness, 188–90
  reflections, 235–37
  safe haven, role of family in, 209–17
  summary of key points, 232–35
  understanding the language of, 227–32

Holmes, Oliver Wendell, Sr. (physician), 324

home, transitioning from work to, 345–47

Hopkins, Adrienne, 367

hospice, 295–96

Hospital Consumer Assessment of Healthcare Providers and Systems (HCAHPS), 7

huddles, group reflection in, 363–65, 377

U

Components of a
Relationship-Based Care Delivery System

The central focus of Relationship-Based Care is the Patient and Family.
All care practices and priorities are organized around
the needs and priorities of patients and families.
Care is experienced when one human being connects with another.

Leaders know the vision, act with purpose, remove barriers, and consistently hold patients, families and staff as their highest priority.

Teamwork requires a group of diverse members from all disciplines and departments to define and embrace a shared purpose and to work together to fulfill that purpose.

Achieving quality outcomes requires planning, precision and perseverance. It begins with defining specific, attainable and measurable outcomes and uses outcome data to continuously enhance performance.

Professional practice integrates compassionate care with clinical knowledge and expertise. Professional nurses work collaboratively with all caregivers, disciplines and departments in the interest of patient care.

Relationship-Based Care

Leadership

Teamwork

Outcomes

Patient & Family

Resources

Professional Practice

Care Delivery

Caring and Healing Environment

A resource driven practice is one which maximizes all available resources, staff, time, equipment, systems and budget.

The patient care delivery system is the infrastructure for organizing and providing care to patients and families. The system determines the way in which the activities of care are accomplished and is built upon the concepts and values of professional nursing practice.

In a caring and healing environment patients, families and colleagues experience care that is attentive to body, mind, and spirit. Caring theory and science informs intentional actions that support self-care, therapeutic relationships with patients, families and healthy peer relationships. Operational practices and physical settings reinforce this commitment to a caring culture.

Relationship-Based Care

(RBC) is an adaptation of Primary Nursing for the current state of health care with short-term patients, part-time nurses, and 12-hour shifts. Relationship-Based Care provides the map and highlights the most direct routes to achieve world-class care and service to patients and families in your organization. Organizations who have implemented this model report an increase in patient satisfaction and loyalty, an increase in staff and physician satisfaction and a more resource conscious and efficient work environment.

Here are some of the ways we can help you implement Relationship-Based Care:

- **Education Session.** How does Relationship-Based Care work on individual units and system wide? What outcomes can be expected? (Half day or one day)

- **Design Day.** A customized design for your organization and the infrastructure needed to support the implementation of the Relationship-Based Care model. (One day)

- **Appreciative Inquiry Organizational Assessment.** Identifies organizational strengths and desired outcomes. (One to two days)

- **Reigniting the Spirit of Caring.** An inspirational/educational experience to enhance awareness about the different dimensions of caring: caring for self, colleagues, patients and their families. (Three days)

- **Leadership at the Point of Care.** Provides clinical leaders the knowledge and skills to create a healing environment for participants and colleagues. (Three days)

- **Relationship-Based Care Practicum.** A practical five day intensive to provide Relationship-Based Care Project Leaders with the clarity and competence essential for assembling a collaborative team of change leaders. Also a chance to share strategies, ideas and challenges with others implementing Relationship-Based Care. (Five days)

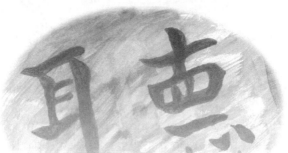

The Therapeutic Relationship Workshop

Being present with another person who is facing trauma, serious illness, loss, and grief requires an awareness and understanding of one's own emotional responses. Only then can the Self be used as a therapeutic tool in the care of others.

This interactive workshop explores the nature of the therapeutic relationship, the conditions under which it can be effective, and the knowledge and skills essential for an authentic human connection to be made in every patient-clinician encounter every time. The workshop focuses on the personal awareness, professional knowledge, and practical and repeatable skills required to see each patient as a person with his or her own unique story and response to the need for care.

This interactive workshop:

- Explores the nature of a therapeutic patient relationship and its value to both the clinician and patient.

- Teaches the self-awareness and practical skills essential for this kind of caregiving response.

In our chaotic and time constrained environments in which technical and complex demands prevail, clinicians struggle as they strive every day to connect with the patients and families in their care. This workshop details specifically how to "see each patient as a person" and not let him or her be made anonymous by the system.

Participants use action learning strategies to practice real-time application and learn guiding principles and a practical methodology that facilitate the clinician's ability to form authentic relationships which improve patient safety and the overall experience of care.

Please visit chcm.com for more information

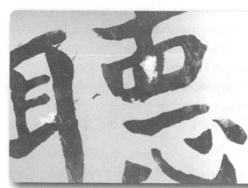

Therapeutic
Relationships

Cultivating personal awareness,
professional knowledge ... and practical
and repeatable skills

Please visit **TheTherapeuticRelationship.com**
*for a discussion of ideas, challenges, issues, and
successes related to therapeutic relationships.*

See Me as a Person: Meditations for Sustaining Relationship-Based Care (RBC)

Michael Trout with Mary Koloroutis

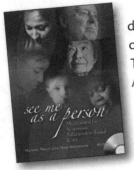

The *See Me as a Person Meditations CD* provides a diverse mix of patient stories and caregiver reflections on therapeutic relationships. Inspired by the Therapeutic Relationships workshop and the book *See Me as a Person: Creating Therapeutic Relationships with Patients and Their Families*, each track is carefully crafted to inspire and deepen the experience of what it means to be fully present for those in our care.

What exactly does reflection have to do with therapeutic relationships? We believe that connection with oneself is a prerequisite to connecting with others. To sustain the capacity for therapeutic relationships, we must stay attuned to our own hearts and minds. As we bring our whole selves to our relationships, a transformation happens on both sides as healing, trust, and mutual respect emerge.

Compact Disc, 63 minutes. (2011) • A520 • $19.95

See Me as a Person Reflection Cards

Mary Koloroutis, Michael Trout

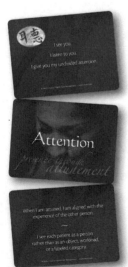

Twenty beautifully designed laminated cards serve as daily reminders to inspire and reinforce therapeutic relationship behaviors and attitudes. Regular use will deepen the experience of creating therapeutic relationships at the point of care. These cards contain everything you want to have front-of-mind when you're about to cross the threshold of the room of a challenging patient or when you've lost touch with the meaning and purpose of your work. These cards, beautifully packaged in an iridescent mesh bag, contain essential language for wondering, following, and holding.

Laminated Card Deck, 20 cards. (2012) • M650 • $14.95

ORDER FORM

1. Call toll-free 800.728.7766 x111 and use Visa, Mastercard or Discover or a company purchase order

2. Fax your order to: 952.854.1866

3. Mail your order with pre-payment or company purchase order to:

    Creative Health Care Management
    5610 Rowland Road, Suite 100
    Minneapolis, MN 55343-8905
    Attn: Resources Department

4. Order Online at: www.chcm.com, click on the "Store" tab.

CREATIVE

HEALTH CARE

MANAGEMENT

Product	Price	Quantity	Subtotal	TOTAL
B650 - See Me as a Person Book	$39.95			
A520CD - See Me as a Person Meditations CD	$19.95			
M650 - See Me as a Person Reflection Cards	$14.95			
B510 - Relationship-Based Care: A Model for Transforming Practice	$34.95			
B560 - I_2E_2: Leading Lasting Change	$24.95			
B558 - What You Accept is What You Teach	$16.00			
Shipping Costs: 1 item = $6.00, 2-9 = $8.00, 10 or more = $10.00 Call for express rates				
Order TOTAL				

Need more than one copy? We have quantity discounts available.

Quantity Discounts		
10–49 = 10% off	50–99 = 20% off	100 or more = 30% off

Payment Methods: ☐ Credit Card   ☐ Check   ☐ Purchase Order PO# _____

Credit Card	Number	Expiration	AVS# (3 digit)
Visa / Mastercard / Discover	– – –	/	
Cardholder address (if different from below):	Signature:		

Customer Information	
Name:	
Title:	
Company:	
Address:	
City, State, Zip:	
Daytime Phone:	
Email:	

Satisfaction guarantee: If you are not satisfied with your purchase, simply return the products within 30 days for a full refund.
For a free catalog of all our products, visit www.chcm.com or call 800.728.7766 x111.